Praise for *Real Kids Real Food Lesson Plans*

"Betsy has addressed a real need in a very comprehensive, easy-to-implement way. I think every parent, teacher, and caretaker of children should take a look at her plan and consider the immense benefits of taking her message to heart and putting it into action. She is a true pioneer!"

—Barbara K. Reid, PhD, MEd, MA, LMFT Chair,
Bachelor of Science in Wellness & Health Promotion Cambridge College

"Lucky are the kids who partake in these classes! Well-thought-out plans with lots of healthy information for all ages."

—Sinéad B.

"I really enjoyed *Real Kids Real Food Lesson Plans* and *Real Kids Real Food Kids-Tested Recipes*. They are refreshing—the ultimate guide to prepare food and have fun at the same time. It encourages kids and their parents to keep exploring and learning about fruit, vegetables, and the healthy lifestyle while exploring the importance of eating healthy, yummy recipes created to be shared with families."

—Celia E.

"The lessons are creative and entertaining for children. They allow kids to learn about food and nutrition in a fun way that is easy to understand."

—Alexia I.

"A beautiful and inspiring pair of books designed to engage kids with delicious and original recipes."

—Mary Alice R.

"The recipes are easy to follow. Listing the benefits of the ingredients is a plus for kids to know, and adults as well."

—Kathleen B.

"Well-illustrated, informative book to present fun and interesting ways to intrigue children to investigate a plant-based diet."

—Kathleen A.

"This book is very impressive in the scope of the lessons and the corresponding activities. A teacher would find this extremely useful in planning a program around healthy eating. The book is full of ideas, activities, and recipes that are yummy and fun!"

—Susana B.

"*Real Kids Real Food Lesson Plans* are thoughtfully prepared with creative ideas that children want to explore. Includes hands-on activities where everyone can participate in their thriving adventures. I really enjoyed the nutritional tips."

—Nancy R.

"*Real Kids Real Food Lesson Plans* provide a clear and easy-to-present set of health values from which all kids can derive great benefit."

—Rob K.

"A perfect guide for any educator to use in teaching kids about developing healthy eating habits. Easy to follow with step-by-step instructions."

—Sally L.

"A healthy lifestyle starts at a young age, and this is the perfect book to teach children how to begin and carry on that journey. The lesson plans and recipes are fun, creative, and simple!"

—Kara L.

"This book is an excellent resource for anyone wanting to teach their children what actual food is. In this day and age, kids don't seem to really know how to eat healthy, and these lessons break it down for them to understand and appreciate high quality, nutritious food."

—Julianna B.

"While *Real Kids Real Food Kids-Tested Recipes* is a rainbow of colors, *Real Kids Real Food Lesson Plans* is a rainbow of information introducing children and adults alike to a healthy lifestyle. Healthy food, exercise, breathing, mindfulness, connection to and respect of nature are all very important to keep our mind and body balanced."

—Valerica S.

"*Real Kids Real Food Lesson Plans* is a valuable book for educators of young children. What fun activities for kids to learn about healthy eating! These easy-to-follow lesson plans are prepared by an experienced teacher and are kid-tested. Kids learn about the nutritional value of a vast number of fruits, vegetables, nuts, seeds and herbs. They also learn about protein, fat, fiber, and carbohydrates, all by getting hands-on experiences of growing and preparing delicious living foods and by learning additional valuable tips for living healthy lives."

—Joy P.

"This book does a wonderful job of teaching children how to eat right from a young age, but does not make this lifestyle seem like a burden at all—to the children or to the parents! It is wonderfully written, easy to follow, and very fun!"

—S. Pearsall

"This book is an excellent companion to the *Real Kids Real Food Kids-Tested Recipes* book. Whether you are a concerned teacher, loving grandmother, or mother, this will fully explain why we eat fresh food and how and why to improve our health on all levels. What a great gift to share with your precious young ones!"

—Cece F.

"I think this is a wonderful opportunity for kids to be introduced to healthy foods at a young age. Usually they are attracted to sweets and junk foods, but this book makes it easy for them to be attracted to healthy, living foods! This is a great book children can even share with their friends and promote healthy living from a young age. Easy read and beautiful pictures."

—Ivone S.

"The words that come to mind are cheery and vibrant. The way the food is presented in this book entices you to want to make the recipes right away! Very colorful and visually appealing."

—Barry H.

"This book is a true gift for any parent or health educator. It presents simple, effective, and proven strategies to teach kids to live healthier and happier lives. A highly-recommended read!"

—Irene Drabkin, Author of *The Power of the Educated Patient*

"Great aid for teachers and parents to help teach children healthy living through diet and lifestyle practices. It's that and more. Appropriate for learners of all ages. Artistic, creative, informative, and highly recommended."

—Eve G.

"Wonderful lessons and recipes to increase children's knowledge of healthy foods and overall health. It's definitely a fun way to get children thinking about healthy options. Great for people of all ages!"

—Margie A.

"This book is full of the wisdom and experience of a lifelong educator, activist, and expert on nutrition whose vision is that of a healthier world. I recommend it to anyone who has children (or doesn't but just wants to be healthier), and especially educators and policy makers who want to learn about and act on ways to benefit our children's health and wellbeing."

—Bruce A.

"This book provides practical lesson plans and recipes for helping teachers and kids learn about healthy eating for a lifetime. Betsy has done a wonderful job of presenting simple, time-tested and fun activities that will allow teachers to immediately incorporate this type of program anywhere!"

—Louise K.

Real Kids Real Food
Lesson Plans

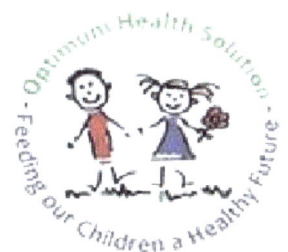

**By Betsy Bragg, Kara Lakin, Leonora Ngo,
Alisha Thapa, and the Real Kids Real Food Team**

Authors
Elizabeth (Betsy) Bragg, Alisha Thapa, Leonora Ngo, and Kara Lakin

Editor
Alisha Thapa and Samantha Finnegan

Cover and Book Design
Leonora Ngo

Photos
FreeDigitalPhotos.net, iStock, Flickr, and Miryam Wiley

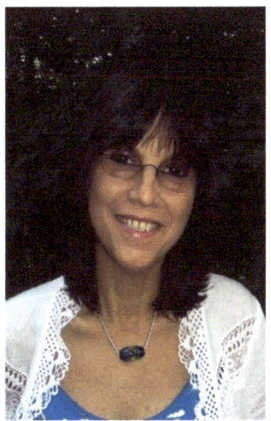

Miryam Wiley

ISBN-13: 978-1534701489
ISBN-10: 1534701486

Table of Contents

Acknowledgements 3

About the Authors 4

Foreword 7

Notes for Use 7

Lesson Plan 1: What is Real Food?...8

Lesson Plan 2: Eating A Rainbow 12

Lesson Plan 3: Eat Local and Seasonal 19

Lesson Plan 4: Sugar Shock...25

Lesson Plan 5: Fruit Art...33

Lesson Plan 6: How to De-stress 36

Lesson Plan 7: Good, Bad, and Ugly Fat 42

Lesson Plan 8: Fabulous Fiber 49

Lesson Plan 9: The Life Cycle of a Plant...55

Lesson Plan 10: Grand Finale 59

Appendix 1: RKRF Physical Activities...63

Appendix 2: Presidential Fitness Program 68

Appendix 3: Jeopardy Questions and Answers 71

Appendix 4: Real Kids Real Food Curriculum 73

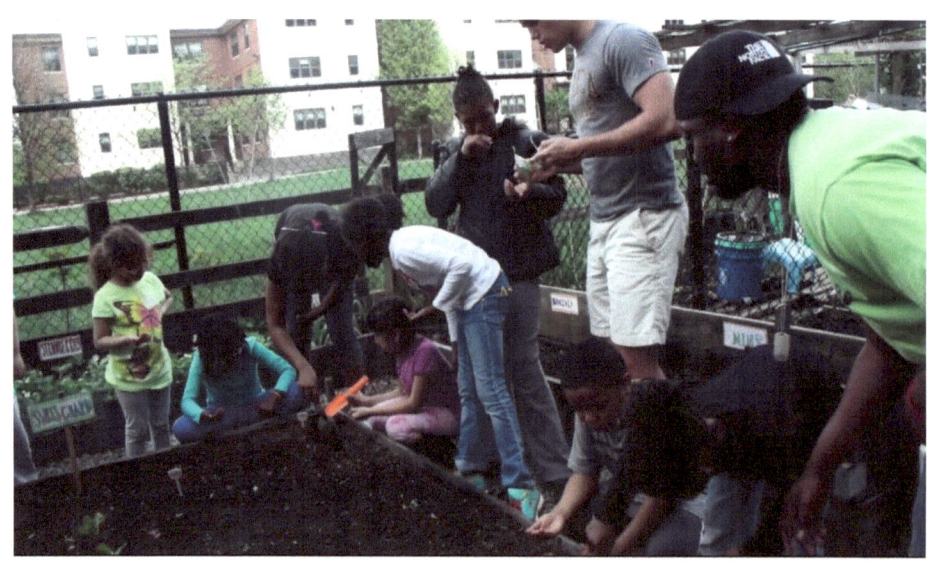

Acknowledgements

We would like to offer special thanks to all the children in the Real Kids Real Food afterschool program at the Mystic Learning Center in Somerville, Massachusetts. We also greatly appreciate the contribution of the staff members, many interns, and passionate volunteers of Real Kids Real Food over the past eight years. We are deeply indebted to the financial supporters that made this program possible: Hippocrates Health Institute, Somerville Health Foundation, eBay Foundation, Ecopolitan Foundation, Allelio Foundation, Sacco Bowling Benefit, Indiegogo Campaign, Kiwanis Club, and several generous anonymous funders. We are deeply indebted to Lisa Brukilacchio, director of Somerville Community Health, and Florence Bergmann for their tremendous support and resources.

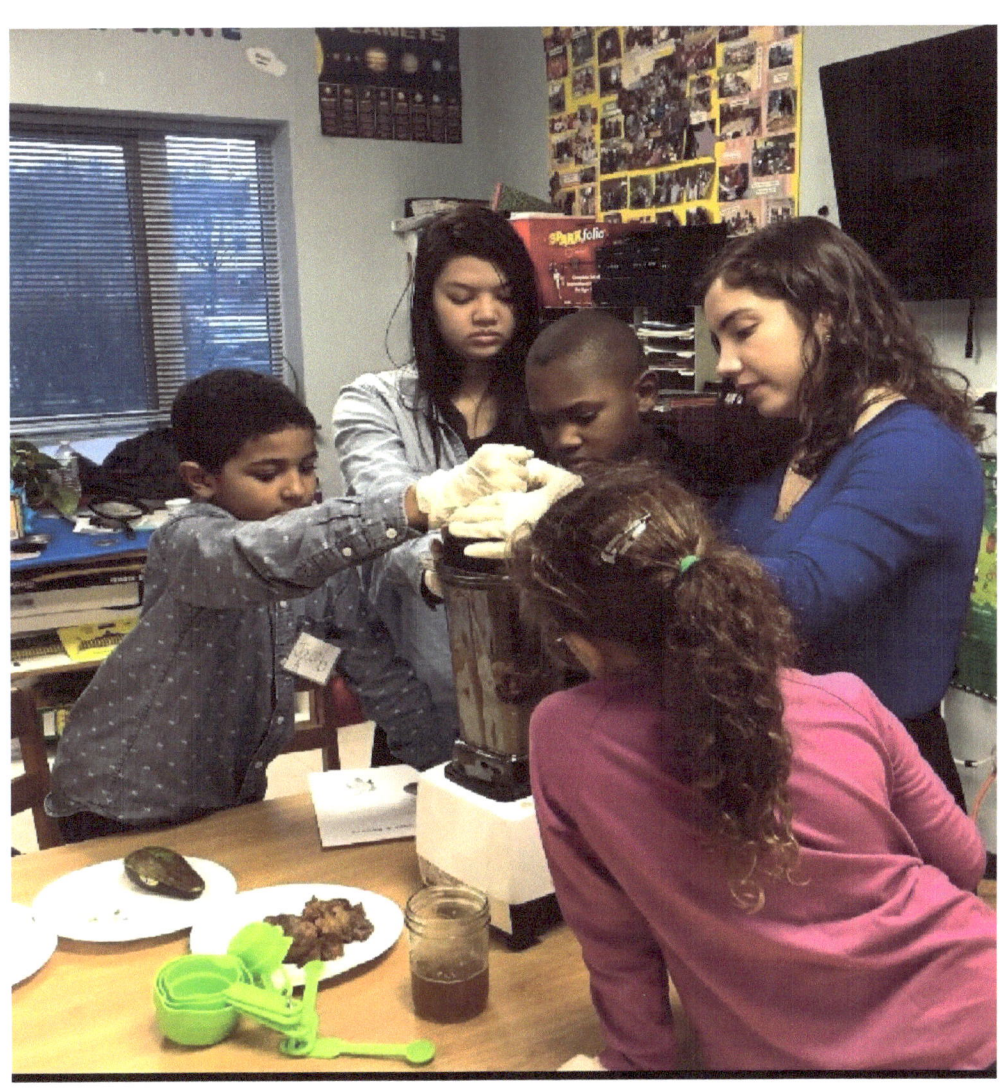

About the Authors

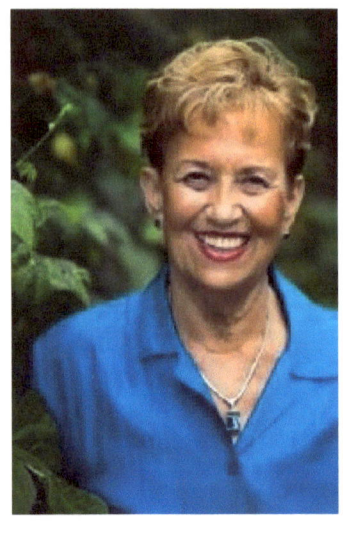

Elizabeth (Betsy) Bragg

Her passion and mission is to prevent obesity, chronic disease, and malnutrition in children through education and advocacy of healthy living. This sprang from her life-changing experiences at the Hippocrates Health Institute (HHI) in West Palm Beach, Florida. Crippled from arthritis and substance abuse, Betsy was gifted by her son a three-week transformational life program at HHI which healed her and inspired her to become certified as an HHI health educator.

Now revitalized at 82 years of age, Betsy is executive director of the nonprofit Optimum Health Solution and founder of Real Kids Real Food, a healthy afterschool program for at-risk, low-income, inner-city children between ages five and twelve.

Betsy's background includes being a director of the Middlesex County Employment and Training Program for Refugees and Immigrants; a teacher from kindergarten through college; and a principal of Lindsley Associates working on economic and social programs with the United Nations, USAID, and Central American Bank in the West Indies, the Philippines, Japan, and El Salvador. She has also worked as a chef, a computer consultant, and a career counselor for students, the unemployed, and the disabled.

Betsy received her bachelor's degree from Smith College in history and English, a master's in counseling and education from Stanford University and Harvard University, a master's in education from Boston University specializing in the administration of multi-cultural non-profit organizations, and a certificate as a Hippocrates Health Educator.

www.OptimumHealthSolution.org; www.RealKidsRealFood.org

Alisha Thapa, Editor

Alisha was the spring 2016 Optimum Health Solution's health educator assistant for the Real Kids Real Food program at the Mystic Valley Learning Center in Somerville, Massachusetts. She is also a public health graduate from Regis College. Her mission is to make a difference in the lives of others by educating and practicing healthy life choices. As a public health major, she strives to promote health and prevent chronic diseases such as diabetes, cardiovascular disease, and obesity.

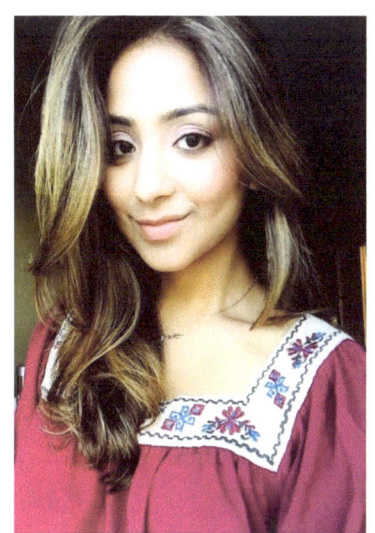

Leonora Ngo, Cover and Book Designer

Over the course of Leonora's internship at Optimum Health Solution as an assistant to the director, she has worked with Betsy Bragg on many projects and fundraising for the Real Kids Real Food program. She graduated from Regis College of Weston, Massachusetts with a degree in public health. Her duties at OHS range from creating slideshows, preparing administrative work, and marketing events, to revising newsletters and updating the website. She also coordinates social media and manages the contact list. Her interest in sustainability is centered on good health and well-being. With her career in public health, she wants to continue to help people of all backgrounds and lifestyles to achieve a healthy, fulfilling life.

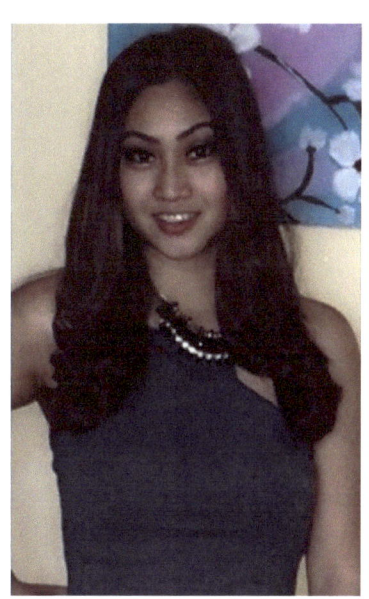

Kara Lakin

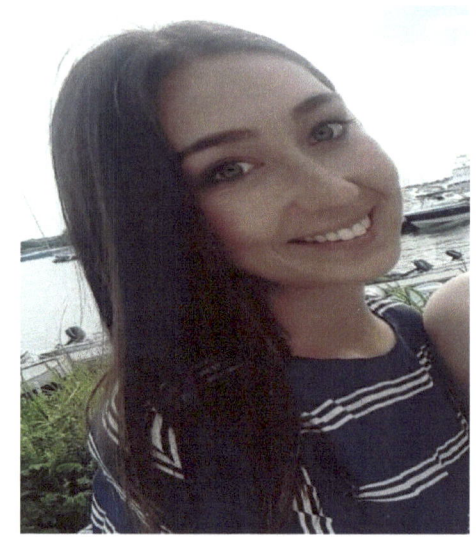

Kara is an assistant intern to the director of Optimum Health Solution. She is a senior at Regis College in Weston, Massachusetts where she majors in health and fitness studies with a concentration in nutrition. She has a passion for nutrition and helping others live more healthfully. With her wide range of knowledge, she has written the teacher and family tips for Real Kids Real Food. When Kara graduates next spring, she plans on attending graduate school to further her career in the nutrition field.

Samantha Finnegan

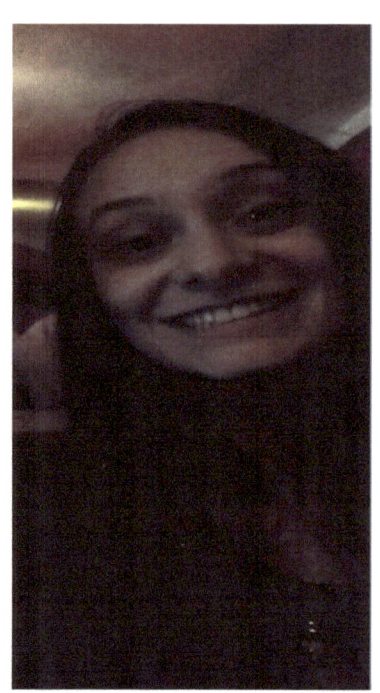

Samantha was the assistant intern to the director of Optimum Health Solution during fall 2016. She is a senior at Regis College in Weston, Massachusetts. She is majoring in nutrition with a minor in public health. With previous experience in the food service industry, she contributed practical ideas and assisted in expanding current events for the program. Upon graduating in the spring, Samantha hopes to attend graduate school and continue helping others to live a healthy, productive life.

Kathy Barrows

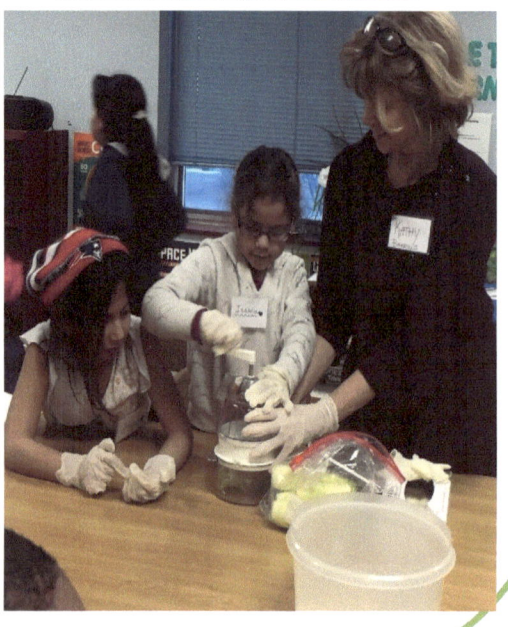

Kathy taught two sessions of Real Kids Real Food at the Mystic Learning Center and at the Benjamin Brown School in Somerville. She has a BS in education with a specialty in recreation therapy from Northeastern University and works as an independent insurance and benefit consultant. She has also earned a certificate in health education from Eat to Thrive. She has a passion for health, wellness, and children, and has volunteered with multiple organizations.

"I learned as much from the children as I hope they learned from me. What a fantastic experience to have such fun while teaching them about making healthier choices."

Foreword

These lesson plans provide comprehensive kid-tested opportunities to learn about healthy food and food preparation through experiential learning.

Embedded in the lessons is also guidance for self-care and well-being skills building, and physical activity to engage the whole child. Tip sheets for teachers and families support on-going learning to reinforce the lessons and add breadth to understanding food and the connections with our health and the wider world. So find a group of kids, prepare the materials as suggested, and get ready to dive into a learning experience that is much broader than just cooking classes. This book will add depth and reflection that will be appreciated by teachers and students alike, enriching your youth development programming!

- Lisa Brukilacchio, OTR/L, MEd, Director of the Somerville Community Health Agenda at Cambridge Health Alliance

Notes for Use

The materials for the recipes in each lesson have been calculated to yield 2-4 ounce servings for 20 individuals. As the size of your class may vary, please consult the recipe to adjust materials as needed.

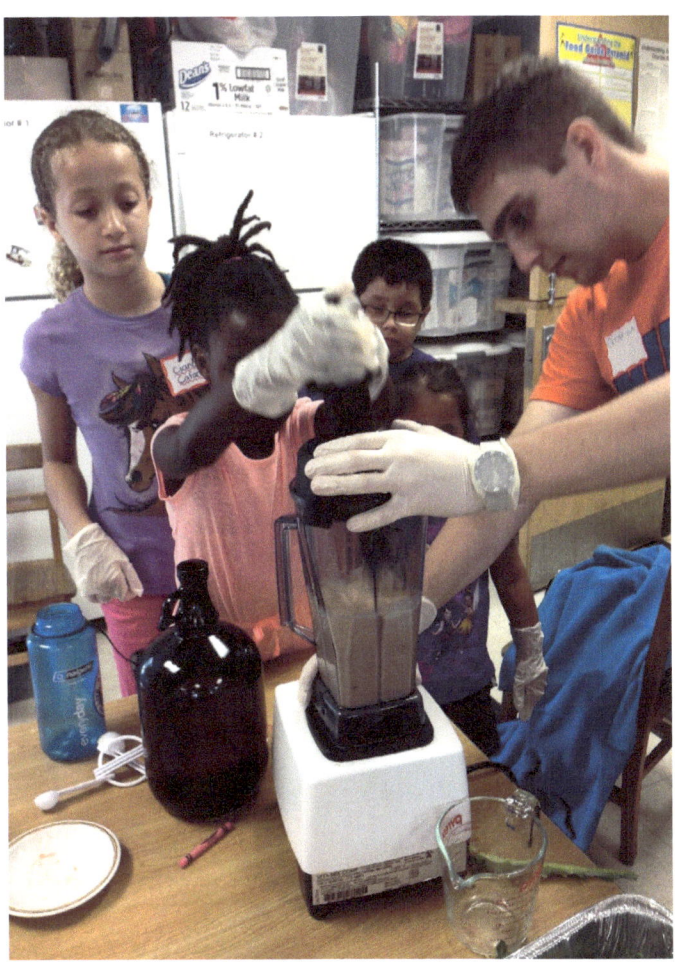

Lesson Plan 1:
What is Real Food?

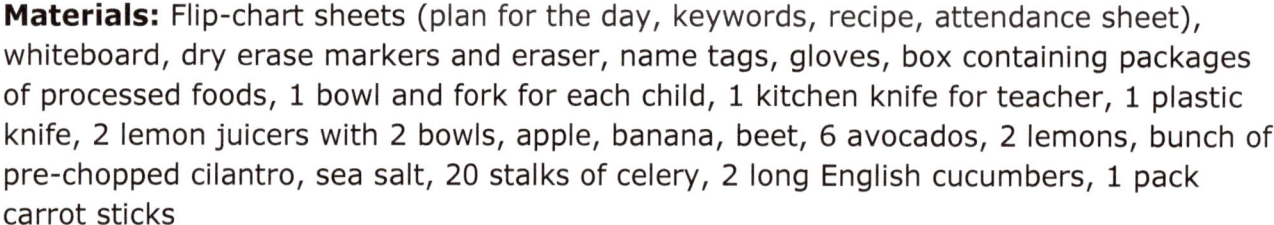

Objectives:
- Introduce Real Kids Real Food
- Understand what real food is
- Be able to differentiate between processed and natural food (bring in examples of each)

Materials: Flip-chart sheets (plan for the day, keywords, recipe, attendance sheet), whiteboard, dry erase markers and eraser, name tags, gloves, box containing packages of processed foods, 1 bowl and fork for each child, 1 kitchen knife for teacher, 1 plastic knife, 2 lemon juicers with 2 bowls, apple, banana, beet, 6 avocados, 2 lemons, bunch of pre-chopped cilantro, sea salt, 20 stalks of celery, 2 long English cucumbers, 1 pack carrot sticks

Plan for the Day

1. Exercise: Land, Sea, Air
This game is for 5 or more people and should be played outside or in an open area. Draw a line on the ground. Pick one person to be the caller. The caller calls out the commands **land**, **sea**, or **air.** If the caller says **land,** everyone jumps behind the line. If the caller says **sea,** everyone jumps over the line. If the caller says **air,** everyone jumps up. If **land** or **sea** is called twice in a row, don't move the second time. If **air** is called twice in a row, jump up both times. If you jump on the line or make a mistake, you're out.

2. Introduction: Show and Tell
Bring a box with a variety of processed food and real food. Go around the classroom and ask each student to identify real food versus processed food.

    a. Nutrition – eating the right kind of food gives strength and energy.
    b. Real food
          i.   Picked – taking it fresh off the tree or ground
          ii. Non-processed – no chemicals added
          iii. Organic – natural and no chemicals added
    c. Processed food – any food that is changed from its natural state

3. Mindfulness: Breathing exercise
Get comfortable, close your eyes, and rest your hands gently on your bellies. First take a deep breath in and a deep breath out. Imagine that your hands are a sailboat, sailing over gently rolling waves. Your breath comes in, your boat gently floats out. The boat does not move on its own. It smoothly bobs up and down with the waves. Take a moment to notice your hands and breathe in this way.

4. Activity: FUNdamentals of food

- Water
  - Makes up 70% of our body/the earth
  - ½ body weight (ounces)
  - Humans can survive one week without water, three weeks without food
  - Body similar to the planet

- Fabulous Fiber
  - Helps your digestion
  - Can help you feel full and keep you from eating too much
  - Examples: celery, chard, apples, whole grains

- Fat
  - Good fats (unsaturated): avocado, nuts (but not peanuts which are legumes that grow in the ground), and seeds
  - Bad fats: from animals, dairy products, canola oil, and many other vegetable oils

- Protein
  - In plants—most in beans, nuts, and seeds

- Carbohydrates
  - What are examples of carbohydrates?
    - Vegetables with the most carbohydrates: potatoes, corn, carrots, beets
  - What are examples of grains?
    - Wheat, quinoa, oats, corn, rye, millet

5. Recipe: Guacamole and Veggies (see page 10)

6. Reflections: Share what they learned without repeating what others say.

Guacamole and Veggies
Servings: 4

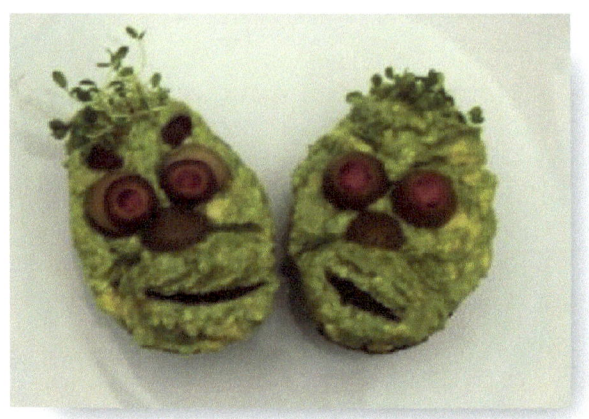

Equipment
Kitchen knife
Plastic knife
Fork for mashing
Lemon juicer
Measuring spoons
Mixing bowl

Ingredients
2 ripe avocados
2 tablespoons chopped fresh cilantro
2 tablespoons lemon juice
Pinch of Celtic sea salt or Himalayan salt
Celery, cucumber, and carrots cut into bite sized pieces

Directions
1. Cut vertically around the entire avocado, then twist the two halves apart.
2. Whack the pit (done by adult) with a kitchen knife, then twist the pit out and discard.
3. Use a plastic knife to dice the avocado halves still in the peel, then scoop out the cubes.
4. Mash the avocado in a bowl.
5. Stir in the remaining ingredients.
6. Serve with celery, cucumber, and carrots for dipping.

Nutrition Tips for Guacamole

Avocados
Cilantro
Lemon Juice

Avocados

Avocados are high in healthy fats. They also have an abundance of nutrients including vitamin K, folate, vitamin C, and potassium—more potassium than bananas! They are loaded with fiber and antioxidants. Avocados are known to help lower cholesterol and triglyceride levels, aid in losing weight, and may help prevent cancer.

Cilantro

Cilantro is a Mediterranean herb that is very low in calories and contains large amounts of antioxidants, vitamins, essential oils, and fiber.

Because of that, cilantro may aid in reducing high cholesterol levels. Cilantro has high traces of potassium, calcium, manganese, iron, and magnesium. Out of all the herbs, it has one of the richest sources of vitamin K.

Lemon Juice

Not only are lemons a super food, but they can also do wonders for any recipe and add so much flavor! The flavonoids in the juice are full of antioxidants. Lemon juice can soothe a sore throat, aid in digestion, support weight loss, bring down a fever, balance out pH levels, and much more!

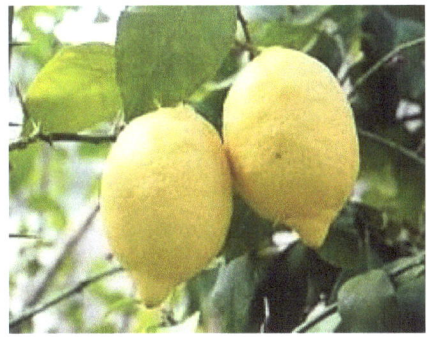
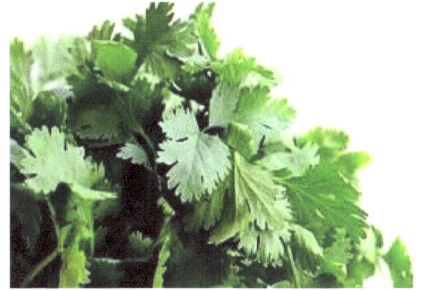

Lesson Plan 2: Eating A Rainbow

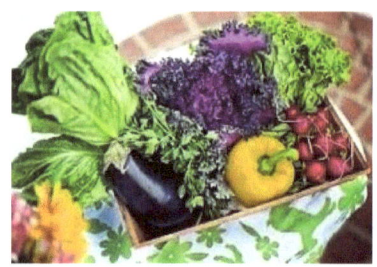 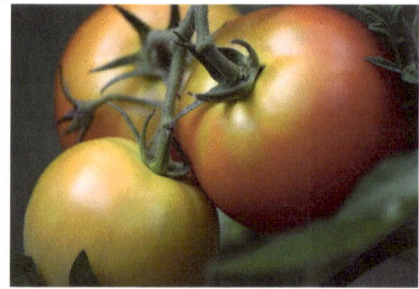

Objectives:
- Learn the nutritional value of different colored fruits and vegetables
- Learn about artificial dyes

Materials: Flip chart sheets (plan for the day, keywords, recipe, attendance sheet), whiteboard, dry erase markers and eraser, name tags, pencils, magic markers, "Eating a Rainbow" coloring charts, 2 blenders, extension cord and power strip, 2 Spiroolis, 2 catching bowls for Spiroolis, serving bowl, measuring cups, 2 sets of measuring spoons, lemon juicer, 1 serving bowl and fork for each child, 12 small or 6 large peeled zucchinis, 16 chopped Roma tomatoes, 8 ounces of sun dried tomatoes (soaked in water for 2 hours), 6 pitted medjool dates, 2 lemons, cold pressed olive oil, dried basil, dried thyme, dried oregano, Himalayan salt

Plan for the Day

1. Exercise: Simon Says

This game is for three or more players. One player takes the role of "Simon" and issues instructions—usually physical actions such as "jump in the air" or "stick out your tongue"—to the other players. Instructions should only be followed if prefaced with the phrase "Simon says." For example: "Simon says touch your nose." If players make a mistake or follow instructions given without the phrase "Simon says," they are out.

2. Mindfulness: One with the Mountain

Get comfortable by sitting in a normal position. Put your hands on your lap or knees. When you are ready, allow your eyes to close, bringing awareness to the breath. Focus on the actual physical sensations, feeling each breath as it comes in and goes out. As you sit here, let an image form in your mind's eye of the most beautiful mountain you have seen or can think of. Continue to focus on it. As you are looking at it, see if you can bring the mountain close to your own body sitting here, so that your body and the mountain in your mind's eye become one. As you sit here, you share in the strength, the stillness, and the majesty of the mountain. You become the mountain. With each breath as you continue sitting, you are becoming a little more like a breathing mountain—alive and vital yet unwavering in your inner stillness; completely what you are, beyond words and thought; a centered, grounded, unmoving presence.

3. Review keywords and last week

a. Nutrition – the process of getting food for your body's health and growth
b. Nutritious – food that is good for you
c. Real food – hand-picked; non-processed; organic
d. Processed – any food that is changed from its natural state
e. Organic – natural, no chemicals added
f. FUNdamentals – water, fiber, protein, carbohydrates, fats and vitamins
g. What percent of your body is water?
h. How much water should you drink? (Ask each child.)

4. Activity: Explain the benefits of each color of fruits and vegetables

- Colors
  i. Red: heart healthy
  ii. Orange/Yellow: protection from some types of cancer; improve night vision
  iii. White: lower cholesterol
  iv. Green: good for bones, teeth, eyes, and preventing diseases such as heart diseases and diabetes
  v. Blue/Purple: improve memory, reduce likelihood of diseases such as cancer, heart diseases, and Alzheimer's

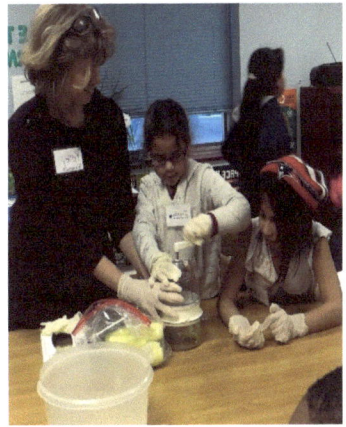

- Activity
  vi. On whiteboard label 5 columns with above colors
  vii. Children list health benefits of each color
  viii. Children list vegetables for each color
  ix. Hand out "Eating a Rainbow" coloring charts with pre-drawn oval broken into five sections
  x. Have each section labeled with a different color and benefit
  xi. Have the children draw the appropriate fruits and vegetables into each section

5. Recipe: Linguini Zucchini with Marinara Sauce (see page 14)

6. Reflection: Share what they learned without repeating what others say.

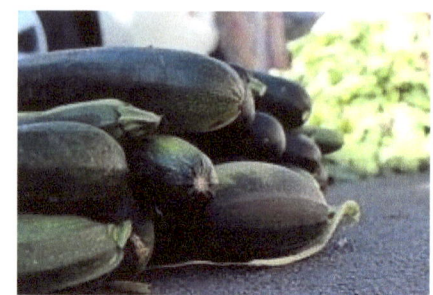

Zucchini Linguini with Marinara Sauce
Prep time: 30 minutes
Servings: 10-12

Equipment
Spirooli
Measuring cups
Measuring spoons
Blender
Large bowl
Lemon juicer

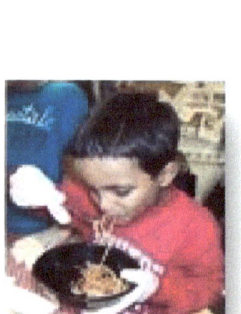

Ingredients for Noodles
6 zucchinis, peeled
3 tablespoons olive oil
3 teaspoons dried basil
1 teaspoon dried oregano
1/2 teaspoon dried thyme

Ingredients for Sauce
8 Roma tomatoes (chopped)
1 cup sun dried (non-oil if possible) tomatoes (soaked for 2 hours; save soaked water)
3 teaspoons dried basil
1 teaspoon dried oregano
1/2 teaspoon dried thyme
2 tablespoons olive oil
3 medjool dates (pitted)
1 tablespoon lemon juice
Salt to taste

Directions
1. Cut ends off zucchini, spiralize, and put in a bowl.
2. Stir 3 tablespoons virgin olive oil, 1 teaspoon oregano, 3 teaspoons basil, and ½ teaspoon thyme together. Toss zucchini in mix to marinate while preparing sauce.
3. Put all sauce ingredients in a blender to combine. If sauce is too thick, thin with water from tomatoes.
4. Pour sauce over noodles, serve, and enjoy.

Nutrition Tips for Zucchini Linguini with Marinara Sauce
Zucchini, Olive Oil, Basil, Oregano, Thyme, Tomatoes, Dates, Lemon Juice

Zucchini
Zucchini is a low-calorie vegetable that has no saturated fat or cholesterol. It is a fantastic source of fiber. Zucchini contains high levels of potassium, which is good for the heart and can lower blood pressure immensely.

Olive Oil
Olive oil is known to be one of the healthiest oils because it contains little saturated fat. It is high in mono-unsaturated fats that help lower bad cholesterol (LDL) and raise good cholesterol (HDL). Foods rich in monounsaturated fatty acids help prevent coronary artery disease and strokes. Make sure it is cold-pressed and in a dark glass bottle.

Basil
Basil's flavonoids and volatile oils both provide numerous health benefits. The flavonoids found in basil protect our cells and fight off unwanted bacterial growth. Basil also has anti-inflammatory effects that can provide relief to health issues such as rheumatoid arthritis or inflammatory bowel conditions.

Oregano
Oregano is made up of plant-based chemical elements that have multiple health benefits. The herb is a rich source of dietary fiber that helps control blood cholesterol levels. Oregano has numerous antioxidants and is an effective antibacterial agent.

Thyme
Like most other herbs, thyme has many health benefits. It has numerous vitamins and minerals that contribute to overall health and wellness. Thyme has antibacterial properties, can lower blood pressure, boost your immunity, boost your mood, help treat acne, and can help stop a cough.

Tomatoes
Tomatoes are known for their high antioxidant levels and their high lycopene content. The combination of the two is extremely good for bone health. Tomatoes have also been shown to be good for your heart as they can lower cholesterol and triglyceride levels. They are high in vitamin C, vitamin K, and biotin.

Dates
Dates are an energy dense fruit that have a high content of natural glucose and fructose. They are an excellent source of dietary fiber. Dates are also rich in potassium, which helps regulate blood pH levels and maintain intracellular fluid balance.

Lemon Juice
Not only are lemons a super food, but they can also do wonders for any recipe and add so much flavor! The flavonoids in the juice are full of antioxidants. Lemon juice can soothe a sore throat, aid in digestion, support weight loss, bring down a fever, balance out pH levels, and much more!

Eating a Rainbow
Teacher Tips

- A sliced **CARROT** looks like the human eye. The cross section of a carrot greatly resembles the pupil, iris, and radiating lines of the human eye—and yes, science shows carrots greatly enhance blood flow to and function of the eyes.

- A **TOMATO** has four chambers and is red just like the heart. Research shows tomatoes are loaded with lycopene which benefits the heart.

- **GRAPES** hang in a cluster that has the shape of a heart. Research shows grapes are also profound heart and blood vitalizing food.

- A **WALNUT** looks like a little brain with left and right hemispheres. Walnuts are good for brain health as well as heart health.

- **KIDNEY BEANS** heal and help maintain kidney functions and look exactly like the human kidney.

- **CELERY** looks like bones and helps to strengthen bones. Celery is 23% sodium and so are bones.

- **AVOCADOS, EGGPLANTS, AND PEARS** are the same shape as a woman's womb and cervix. Like babies in the womb, avocados take 9 months to grow. When a woman eats one avocado a week it can help prevent cervical cancer.

- **SWEET POTATOES** look like and increase the health of the pancreas.

- **OLIVES** look like and increase the health of the ovaries.

- **GREEN** produce lowers the risk of some cancers and supports vision health and the growth of strong bones and teeth. Some examples of green foods are avocados, green apples, limes, honeydew, kiwi, artichokes, asparagus, broccoli, cabbage, green beans, peas, and zucchinis.

- **WHITE** foods lower the risk of some cancers, promote heart health, and maintain cholesterol levels that are already healthy. This includes bananas, cauliflower, garlic, ginger, jicama, mushrooms, and white corn.

- **YELLOW/ORANGE** foods lower the risk of some cancers, support heart and vision health, and promote a healthy immune system. Apricots, cantaloupes, grapefruit, mangoes, nectarines, oranges, pineapples, squash, carrots, yellow peppers, pumpkin, and sweet potatoes are some common examples.

- **RED** foods lower the risk of some cancers and support heart, memory, and urinary tract health. Includes foods like red apples, strawberries, watermelon, beets, red peppers, radishes, red onions, and tomatoes.

- **BLUE/PURPLE** foods lower the risk of some cancers, maintain urinary tract health, support memory function, and lead to healthy aging. Some common blue/purple foods include blackberries, blueberries, raisins, grapes, prunes, and eggplant.

Rainbow Charts

List fruits and veggies of each color in the appropriate column.

GREEN	WHITE	RED	YELLOW	BLUE
Kiwi	Bananas	Cranberries	Mangoes	Blueberries
Asparagus	Brown pears	Radishes	Squash	Blackberries
Cucumbers	Cauliflower	Red peppers	Peaches	Grapes
Green apples	Ginger	Rhubarb	Papaya	Raisins
Peas	Garlic	Tomatoes	Yellow apples	Plums
Zucchini	Mushrooms	Watermelon	Pineapples	Eggplant
Cabbage	Dates	Grapefruit	Sweet corn	Prunes
Green beans	White corn	Red apples	Lemon	
Leafy greens	Potatoes	Strawberries	Cantaloupe	
Honeydew	White peaches	Pomegranates	Yellow peppers	
Celery	White nectarines	Raspberries	Apricots	
Brussels sprouts	Onions	Cherries	Butternut squash	
Broccoli	Turnips	Beets		
Green onion	Shallots	Red onion		
Spinach				
Limes				
Avocados				
Watercress				

Eat Your Colors
Family Tip Sheet

Today your child learned...

- Eating at least 5 servings of colorful fruits and vegetables each day helps us grow and be strong.

- Adding color to your diet is a fun and tasty way to add variety.

- Healthy snacks are an important part of your diet. The healthiest snacks contain fruits and vegetables in combination with low fat dairy, whole grains, or proteins.

Why is this important?

- Eating fruits and vegetables of different colors gives you a wide range of vitamins, minerals, fiber, and other chemicals that your body needs to stay healthy and fight off disease.

- The variety of colors maximizes the nutritional benefits.

Here's what you can do:

- Feed your family a variety of fruits and vegetables each day.

- Try one new fruit and one new vegetable each week.

- The next time you're at the grocery store, let your child/children pick out a new fruit or vegetable to try.

- Try to make meals and snacks as colorful as possible.

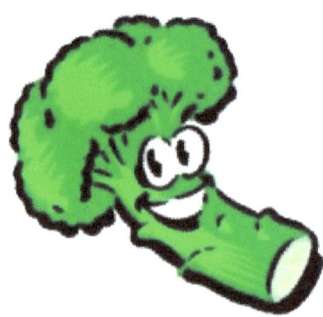

Lesson Plan 3: Eat Local and Seasonal

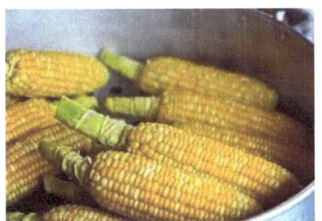

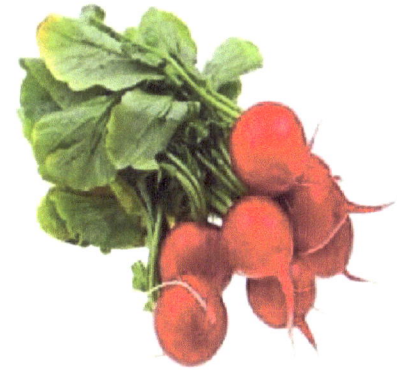

Objective: Eat local and seasonal for sustainability

Materials: Flip-chart sheets (plan for the day, keywords, recipes, attendance sheet), whiteboard, dry erase markers and eraser, name tags, vegetable peeler, 2 kitchen knives, 2 measuring cups, measuring spoons, 4 cutting boards, 2 blenders, carafe, tablecloth, 1 bowl and spoon per child, 5 sweet potatoes, 5 avocados, 5 tablespoons tamari, 5 knobs of ginger roots, Himalayan salt, ground black pepper, electric kettle, 2 quarts of water, 2 (16 ounce) bags of frozen organic corn, 1 leek

Plan for the Day

1. Exercise: Jump Rope Challenge
Two people hold either end of the jump rope and swing the rope in the same direction. Children will try to jump in and over the rope, taking one or two jumps before safely exiting the swinging rope. When a child fails to join in, jump over, or exit the swinging rope (interrupting the swings), he or she is out until the next round.

2. Mindfulness: Muscle relaxation
Sit in a comfortable chair or lie on your back. Rest your hands at your sides and close your eyes. Take a deep breath and let it out with a sigh. Let your body relax as you release your breath. Feel your chest and shoulders rising up slightly as you breathe in, then dropping and relaxing as you breathe out. With every breath, breathe away some of your stress. The simple act of breathing can allow you to slow down and start to relax. Focus on your body, noticing how your body feels right now. However you are feeling, good or bad, is okay. Just observe how your body feels without trying to change anything yet.

Raise your shoulders up toward your ears and tighten your muscles. Hold and feel the tension there before you release. Let your shoulders drop to a lower, more comfortable position. Tighten your hands into fists—very, very tight as if you are squeezing a rubber ball very tightly in each hand. Feel the tension in your hands and forearms, then release. Shake your hands gently, shaking out the tension. Feel how much more relaxed your hands are now. Breathe in deeply and hold that breath. Feel the tension as you hold the air in. Hold, then relax. Let the air be released through your mouth. Breathe out all the air.

3. Introduction: Keywords
- Local
- Seasonal

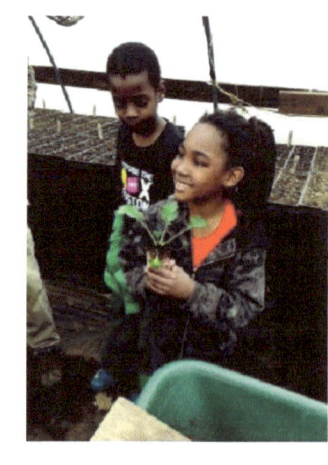

4. **Activity:** Seasonal and local fruits and vegetables
- Explain why we eat certain vegetables in certain seasons
- Fall: squash, corn, pumpkins, apples
- Year-round: kale

5. **Recipe:** Corn and Sweet Potato Chowder (see page 21)

6. **Reflection:** Share what they learned without repeating what others say.

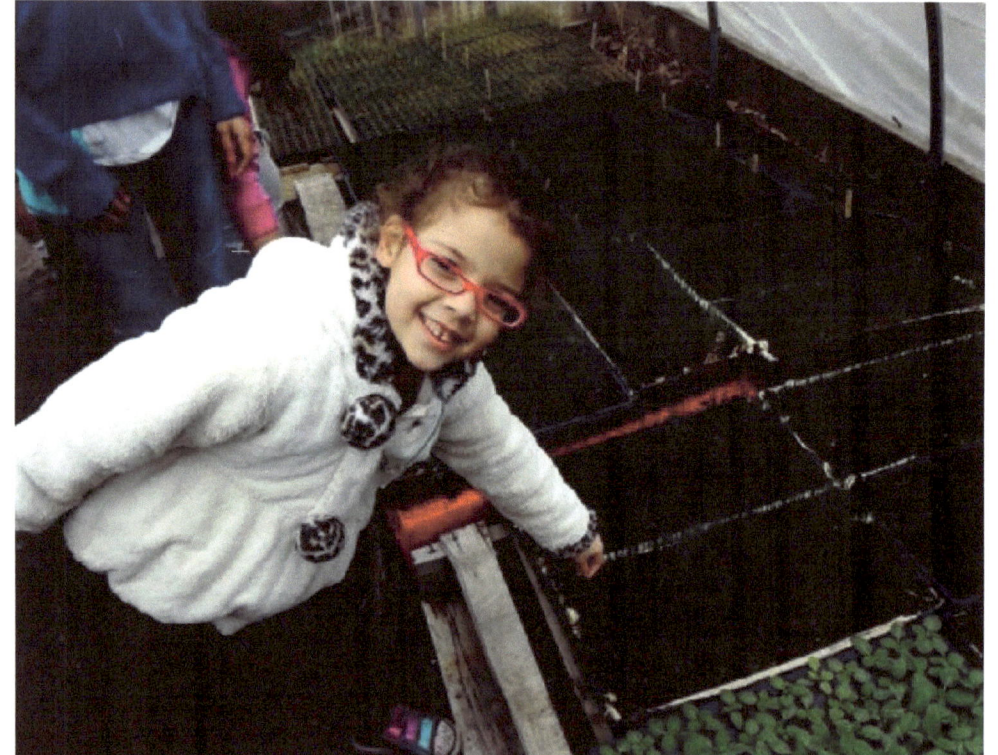

Corn and Sweet Potato Chowder
Servings: 4

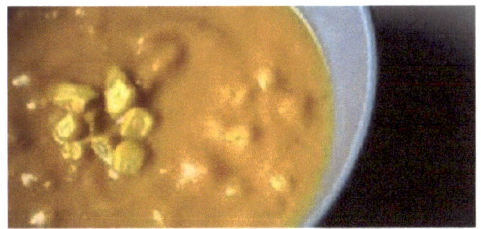

Equipment

Measuring cups
Measuring spoons
Kitchen knife
Cutting board
Electric kettle
Blender
Peeler

Ingredients

1 cup sweet potato
1 whole avocado
1 tablespoon miso tamari
1 small knob of ginger, peeled and finely chopped
½ cup roughly chopped leek
dash of salt
dash of pepper
1 cup hot water
2 cups frozen organic corn

Directions

1. Peel and cut sweet potato and ginger.
2. Place all the ingredients except for the corn in a blender and blend until the texture is smooth.
3. Taste and adjust seasoning if necessary.
4. Remove from the blender and put into a bowl with the corn.

Nutrition Tips for Corn and Sweet Potato Chowder

Sweet Potatoes

Avocados

Miso Tamari

Ginger

Corn

Sweet Potatoes

Many people do not realize all of the health benefits that sweet potatoes have. They are full of antioxidants, anti-inflammatory nutrients, and blood sugar-regulating nutrients. Sweet potatoes have very high concentrations of vitamin A, vitamin C, and manganese.

Avocados

Avocados are high in healthy fats. They also have an abundance of nutrients including vitamin K, folate, vitamin C, and potassium—more potassium than bananas! They are loaded with fiber and antioxidants. Avocados are known to help lower cholesterol and triglyceride levels, aid in losing weight, and may help prevent cancer.

Miso Tamari

Tamari is often used as a substitute for salt in cooking. It has great flavor! It is often considered the healthy version of soy sauce. While soy sauce is made with wheat, tamari contains little to no wheat. Tamari is full of antioxidant and anti-cancer properties.

Ginger

Ginger is one of the healthiest spices on earth. It is made up of gingerol, which is a potent substance with multiple medicinal properties. It can reduce nausea and muscle pain, lower blood sugar, treat indigestion, reduce menstrual pain, lower cholesterol levels, and much more.

Corn

Whole grain corn is rich in fiber along with a variety of vitamins, minerals, and antioxidants. Corn is made up mostly of carbohydrates but has small amounts of fat and protein as well. It also contains phytochemicals that protect against numerous chronic diseases.

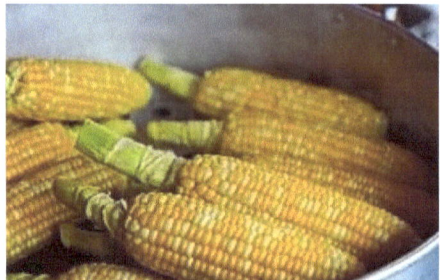
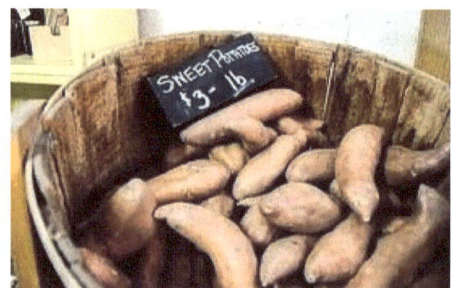

Eat Local and Seasonal
Family Tip Sheet

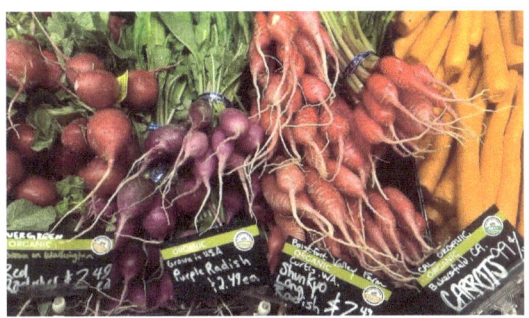

Why should your family eat local and seasonal?

- Eating a diet that follows nature's patterns is the best way to lead a healthy lifestyle and improve nutrition.

- Not only do fruits and vegetables reach their nutritional peak when they need to be harvested, but they also reach their flavor peak as well.

- Eating locally and seasonally is more affordable and is better for your community's economy.

What fruits and vegetables are in season?

Winter: bananas, beets, brussels sprouts, cabbage, carrots, grapefruit, kale, lemons, onions, oranges, pears, sweet potatoes, turnips

Spring: apricots, asparagus, apples, broccoli, collard greens, garlic, lettuce, mushrooms, peas, radishes, spinach, strawberries, swiss chard

Summer: bell peppers, blackberries, blueberries, cantaloupe, cherries, corn, eggplant, green beans, kiwi, mangos, peaches, cucumbers, okra

Fall: cauliflower, cranberries, ginger, grapes, onions, parsnips, pineapple, potatoes, pumpkins, radishes, spinach, rutabagas, and raspberries

How to make it fun for your kids!

- Take them to the farmers' market and let them pick out seasonal fruit and vegetables. They can even weigh their items.

- Try samples. Booths at farmers' markets will often have samples set out for customers to try. This is a good way to get your children to try new things!

- Prepare and cook foods using your farmers' market purchases.

Eat Local and Seasonal
Teacher Tips

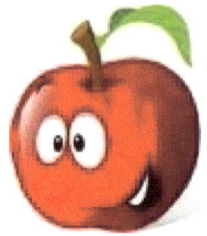

Why do we eat certain vegetables and fruits in certain seasons?

When you eat in season, you are in tune with nature and it's healthier. You also get the most flavor and nutritional value, in addition to it being more affordable.

Fall vegetables and fruits: Why are they good for us?
- Squash – Squash is important for our vision and bone growth, protects our heart, and keeps us strong.
- Corn – Corn is a rich source of fiber. It is important for our digestive system; it has vitamins A, B, and E, and many minerals.
- Apples – Apples are a great source of fiber. They also have vitamin C and calcium which help to build a strong body.
- Pumpkins – Pumpkins help our brain function, promote healthy skin, keep eyesight sharp, boost our immune system, and help with weight loss.

Why eat local?
- Local is fresher, healthier, and tastes better.
- Local uses less fuel to get to the markets.
- Local builds relationships between the consumers and the farmers.

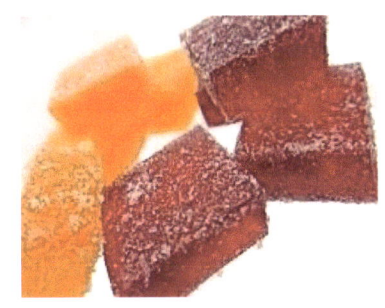

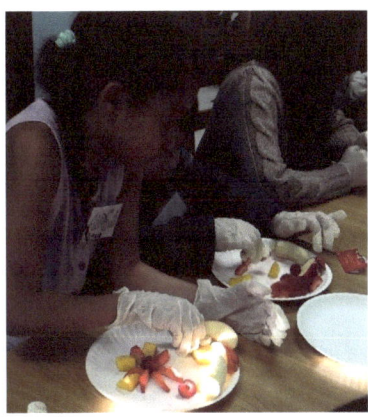

Lesson Plan 4: Sugar Shock

Objectives:
- Learn how sugar affects the body and how we can minimize/substitute our intake
- Learn the amount of sugar in different drinks

Materials: Flip-chart sheets (plan for the day, keywords, recipe, attendance sheet), whiteboard, dry erase markers and eraser, name tags, Sugar Shock worksheets, markers, pencils, 1 bowl and spoon per child, latex gloves, 2 blenders, extension cord and power strip, 1 tablecloth, 4 cutting boards, 4 apple slicers, 2 sets of measuring spoons, 1 kitchen knife, 3 lemon juicers, 2 large bowls, 2 spatulas, 2 serving spoons, 20 apples, 8 medjool dates, 3 lemons, cinnamon, 14 8-ounce glass jars, sugar, empty bottles of each of the following: apple juice, Coca-Cola, Sprite, root beer, Gatorade, orange juice, skim milk, chocolate milk, whole milk, lemonade, ginger ale, iced tea, energy drink, water

Plan for the Day

1. Exercise: Popper Stomper
Stomp the other balloons but watch out for yours! Players tie a string to the end of a balloon and then tie it around one of their ankles. Then players run around trying to pop each other's balloons without getting their own popped. The game works better if the playing field is on the smaller side so that players can't run too far away.

2. Mindfulness: Peaceful Meadow
Take a moment to relax your body. Get comfortable. Notice how your body feels, and make some slight adjustments to increase your comfort. Take a deep breath in. Hold it and breathe out, releasing your tension. Imagine yourself walking outdoors. You are walking through the trees—small aspens, their leaves moving in a slight breeze. The sun shines down warmly. You walk toward a clearing in the trees. As you come closer to the clearing, you see that it is a meadow. You walk out of the trees, into the meadow. Tall green grass blows gently. You are probably feeling a bit tired. It would be so nice to sit down in the grass. Feel the breeze caress your skin as you sit or lie down in the sun. It is a pleasant day, warm but not hot, quiet and peaceful.

3. Key Words
- Sugar – sweet substance usually in the form of white or brown crystals that comes from plants and is also manufactured from chemicals.
- Carbohydrate – good carbs are found in natural fruits, vegetables and grains. Bad carbs come from processed foods like candy, cake, ice cream, and sodas. They provide your body with heat and energy.
- Diabetes – a serious disease in which the body cannot properly control the amount of sugar in your blood because it does not have enough insulin (a substance that your body makes and uses to turn sugar into energy).
- 4 grams = 1 teaspoon of sugar

4. Activity: Sugar Shock worksheet (see page 29)
- Have children choose their 5 favorite drinks and circle them.
- Children will then guess the number of teaspoons of sugar in each drink and write that number down.
- Once they have guessed, show them the answer sheet and have them write down the correct answer.
- One child at a time reads the amount of sugar on the label and all children look for the glass jar that contains the corresponding amount of sugar and puts it next to the bottle.
- Children line up all the empty bottles in the middle of the table from least to most amount of sugar.

5. Recipe: Applesauce (see page 27)

6. Reflection: Share what they learned without repeating what others say.

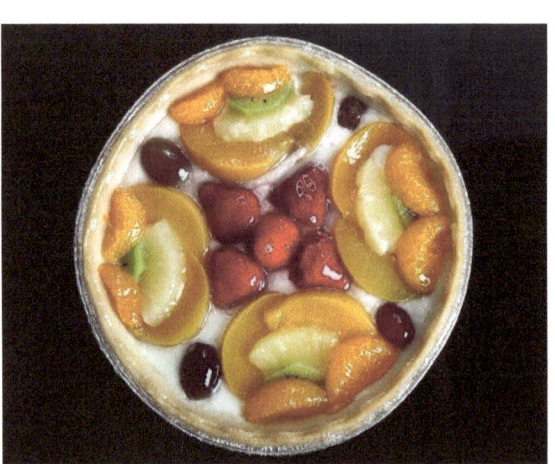

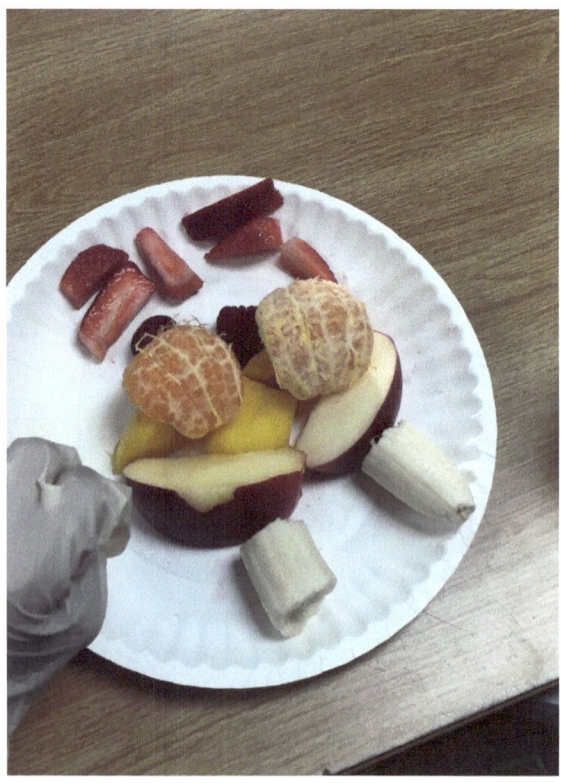

Applesauce
Servings: 4

Equipment
Cutting board
Kitchen knife
Blender
Lemon juicer
Bowl

Ingredients
4 apples
2 medjool dates, pitted, soaked for 2 hours
1 tablespoon lemon juice
Ground cinnamon

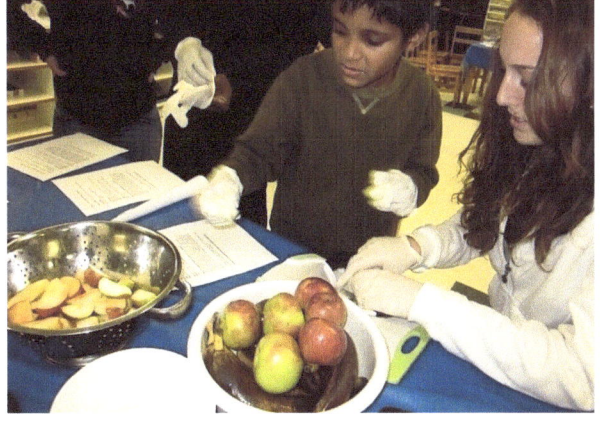

Directions
1. Cut apples into slices then place in a blender.
2. Add medjool dates and lemon juice and blend again.
3. Sprinkle in a little cinnamon and blend one last time. Pour into a large bowl to serve and enjoy!

Fun Fact: There are thousands of different varieties of apples including fuji, gala, red delicious, golden delicious, pink lady, and granny smith.

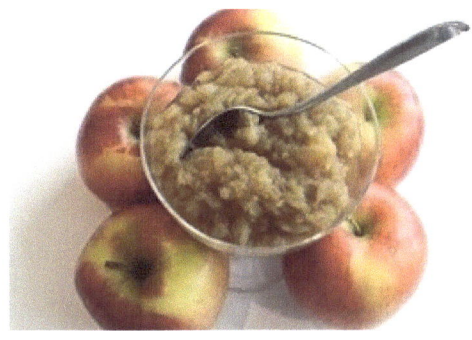

Nutrition Tips for Applesauce
Apples
Medjool Dates
Lemon Juice
Cinnamon

Apples
Apples are full of phytonutrients that can aid in regulating your blood sugar levels. Apples also have high amounts of fiber. Eating a diet high in fiber has many health benefits including reducing the risk of certain diseases, controlling blood sugar and blood fat levels, and maintaining your digestive tract.

Medjool Dates
Dates are an energy-dense fruit that have a high content of natural glucose and fructose. Like apples, they are an excellent source of dietary fiber which provides numerous health benefits. Dates are also rich in potassium, which helps regulate blood pH levels and maintain intracellular fluid balance.

Lemon Juice
The benefits of lemons are endless. Lemon juice is an excellent source of vitamin C, can help relieve indigestion and constipation, is used in skin care and weight loss, can be used to treat respiratory disorders and rheumatism, balance pH levels, and even flush out toxins.

Cinnamon
Cinnamon is a potent antioxidant that has various health benefits. It has anti-inflammatory compounds that can boost brain function, boost immunity, lower bad cholesterol, and regulate blood sugar.

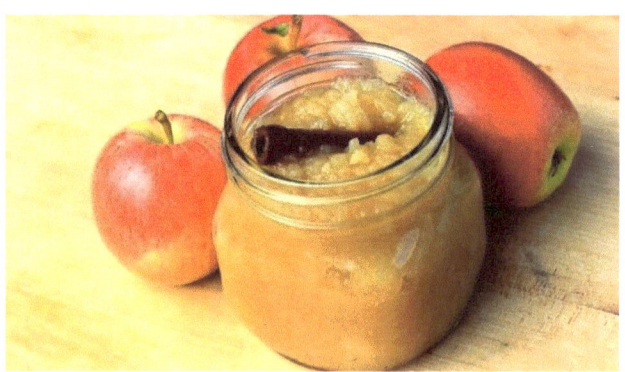

Sugar Shock
What are your favorite drinks?

Instructions: Choose your 5 favorite drinks and circle them. Then guess the number of teaspoons of sugar in each drink and write that number down. Assume that soft drinks are a 12-fl. oz. can and other drinks are an 8-fl. oz. cup/bottle. (Remember: 4 grams makes 1 teaspoon!)

Drink	# of teaspoons of sugar
Apple Juice	_____
Coca-Cola	_____
Sprite	_____
Root Beer	_____
Gatorade	_____
Orange Juice	_____
Skim Milk	_____
Chocolate Milk	_____
Whole Milk	_____
Lemonade	_____
Ginger Ale	_____
Iced Tea	_____
Energy Drink	_____
Water	_____

Sugar Shock Activity Kit

Directions for creating the kit: For the Sugar Shock activity, children will learn how much sugar is in drinks on the market. Collect the following empty drink bottles, containers, and cans and the corresponding number of 8-ounce jars. Fill each jar with the amount of sugar listed on each drink container. Paste labels on each jar with the amount of sugar in grams and teaspoons. With this information, a kit can be created for your own class. This kit can be kept in a small box or suitcase

Materials: Empty drink bottles, jars, sugar

Drink	# of teaspoons of sugar	# of grams of sugar
Apple Juice	7	28
Chocolate Milk	6	24
Coca-Cola	10	40
Energy Drink	9	36
Gatorade	4	16
Ginger Ale	9	36
Iced Tea	9	36
Lemonade	7	28
Orange Juice	5	20
Root Beer	7	14
Skim Milk	3	12
Sprite	9	36
Water	0	0
Whole Milk	3	12

Sugar Shock
Teacher Tips

How much sugar do we consume each day?
- In the US, an average child between 7 and 14 years old consumes 21 teaspoons of sugar each day, which is half a cup.
- The average child under the age of 12 consumes 49 pounds of sugar per year.
- To be healthy, children ages 4 to 12 should only eat 3 teaspoons of sugar a day.

What happens when we eat sugar?
- Sugar makes us hyper and then makes us feel tired and sluggish.
- When sugar enters the bloodstream and reaches the brain, it temporarily increases calming neurochemicals such as serotonin.
- Drinking even one sugary drink a day often leads to:
    - Unhealthy weight gain
    - Obesity
    - Diabetes
    - Chronic heart diseases
    - Tooth decay/cavities

Informational Notes: Diabetes

- **What is diabetes?** Diabetes is a chronic condition where there is too much glucose (sugar) in the blood. There is a hormone in our body called insulin which is made in the pancreas and allows the sugar in our bloodstream to enter our cells and be used for energy. If our body does not produce enough insulin or the insulin can't reach our cells, sugar levels in the bloodstream rise and diabetes occurs. [1]
- **Types of diabetes:** Most commonly, children have type 1 diabetes. This occurs when the pancreas is not able to create enough insulin. Type 2 diabetes usually occurs in adults, but is being diagnosed in children with increasing frequency. In type 2 diabetes the pancreas still creates insulin but not effectively.[1]
- **Symptoms:** Symptoms of both type 1 and type 2 diabetes include increased thirst, increased urination, fatigue, hunger, and blurry vision. [2]
- **Causes:** Genetics and lifestyle both play important roles in the cause of diabetes.
- **Statistics:** Diabetes remains the seventh leading cause of death in the United States. Approximately 1.25 million American adults and children have type 1 diabetes. [3]

[1] "Diabetes & Kids," 2016, http://www.diabetesresearch.org/document.doc?id=274
[2] "Diabetes Symptoms," 2014, http://www.healthline.com/health/diabetes-symptoms#Overview1
[3] "Statistics About Diabetes," 2016, http://www.diabetes.org/diabetes-basics/statistics/

Avoid Sugary Food
Family Tip Sheet

Do you know how much sugar your child eats?

- In the US, an average child between 7 and 14 years old consumes 21 teaspoons of sugar each day, which is half a cup.
- The average child under the age of 12 consumes 49 pounds of sugar per year.
- To be healthy, children ages 4 to 12 should only eat 3 teaspoons of sugar a day.

Eating too much of sugar can put your kids at risk of:

- Hyperactivity
- Gaining excess weight
- Diabetes
- High blood pressure
- High cholesterol
- Chronic heart disease

Easy tips to avoid sugary food for your kids:

- Sugar should not be in the first 5 items on the nutrition label. Keep in mind that 4 grams is about 1 teaspoon.
- Avoid processed foods.
- Avoid added sugar, corn syrup, dextrose, fructose, and other sweeteners.
- Skip sodas and processed juices.

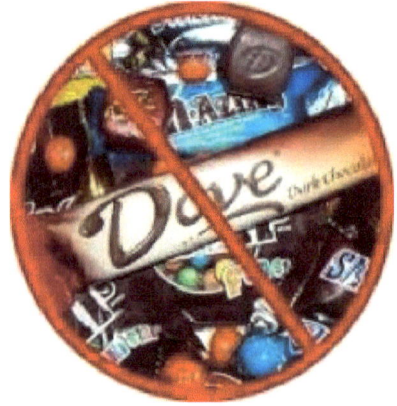 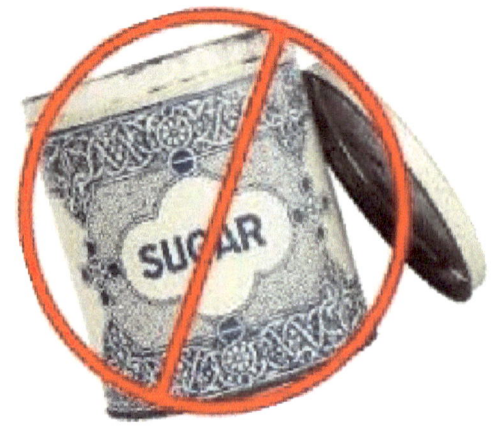

Lesson Plan 5: Fruit Art

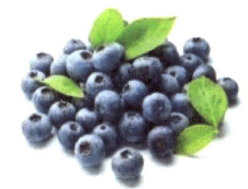

Objectives:
- Fun with real food
- Review what we've learned

Materials: Flip-chart sheets (plan for the day, keywords, recipe, attendance sheet), whiteboard, dry erase markers and eraser, name tags, hula hoop, Jeopardy board, extension cord and power strip, fruit stickers, 2 kitchen knives, 4 cutting boards, 4 apple slicers, plastic knives, 2 blenders, 2 extra carafes, tablecloth, 1 paper plate and cup per child, gloves, 4 apples, 4 mangoes, 10 bananas, 1 quart strawberries, 6 clementines, ½ pint raspberries, 1 cup shredded coconut, 1 quart water

Plan for the Day

1. Exercise: Hula Hoop Relay Race

Divide group into two teams. The players on each team join hands to form a line. Loop a hula hoop over one player's arm. Without letting go of the other players' hands, he or she must step into and through the hoop so it rests on his or her other arm then slide it onto the next player's arm so he or she can repeat the same maneuver. Whichever team can pass the hoop to the front of the line and back first without letting go of each other's hands is the winner. Winning team gets fruit stickers.

2. Mindfulness

To begin, lie down and make yourself comfortable. Start becoming aware of your breathing. Notice each breath as it goes in and out. Take a moment to focus your attention on your breathing without trying to change anything. Just notice your breathing, focusing intently on each breath. As you relax, start to create a picture in your mind. Imagine that you are lying on a blanket outside on a warm summer day. The blanket is in the soft grass next to some trees. The sun shines down warmly and a cool breeze blows across your skin. See the sky above, blue and bright. See the clouds floating by, blowing in the breeze. Picture in your mind the details of this scene. Feel the sun and breeze on your skin, feel the soft grass and blanket beneath you. Watch the clouds passing the branches as they drift by. Notice the different shapes of clouds. Some are round, fluffy cumulus clouds. Others are long, thin, wispy clouds like streaks of semi-transparent white paint across the blue of the sky. The clouds drift lazily by, slowly, smoothly floating.

3. Jeopardy Review Game (see page 71)

4. Activity: Fruit Art

On a paper plate, make a face or design using 1 strawberry cut in quarters, 3 raspberries, 5 pieces of mango, 3 pieces of clementine, ½ banana, 3 slices of apple, and 1 tablespoon of shredded coconut. Pass out only these quantities to each. Take photos.

5. Recipe: Fruit Art Smoothie (see page 34)

6. Reflections: Share what they learned without repeating what others say.

33

Fruit Art Smoothie
Servings: 4

Equipment
Cutting board

Kitchen knife

Blender

Paper cups

Ingredients
2 frozen bananas

1/3 mango

1/3 apple

3 clementines

1/3 cup of raspberries

2 tablespoons shredded coconut

1/3 cup water

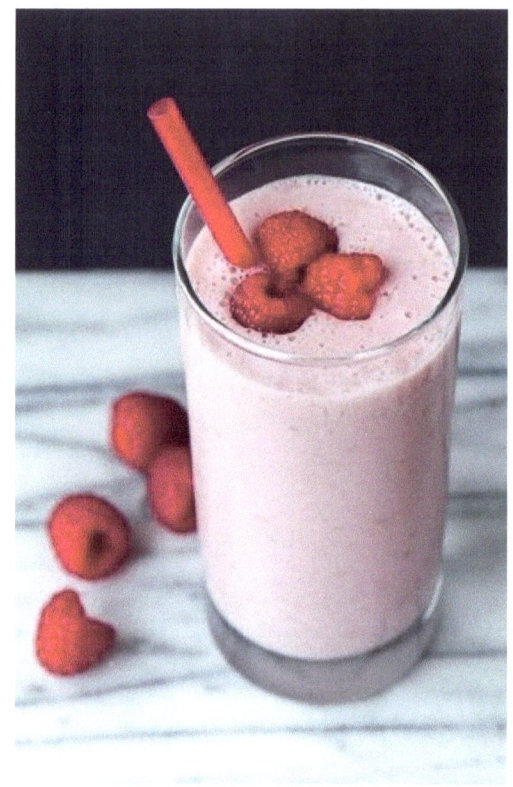

Directions
1. Combine fruit in blender.
2. Use water to thin smoothies to desired consistency.
3. Serve in paper cups.

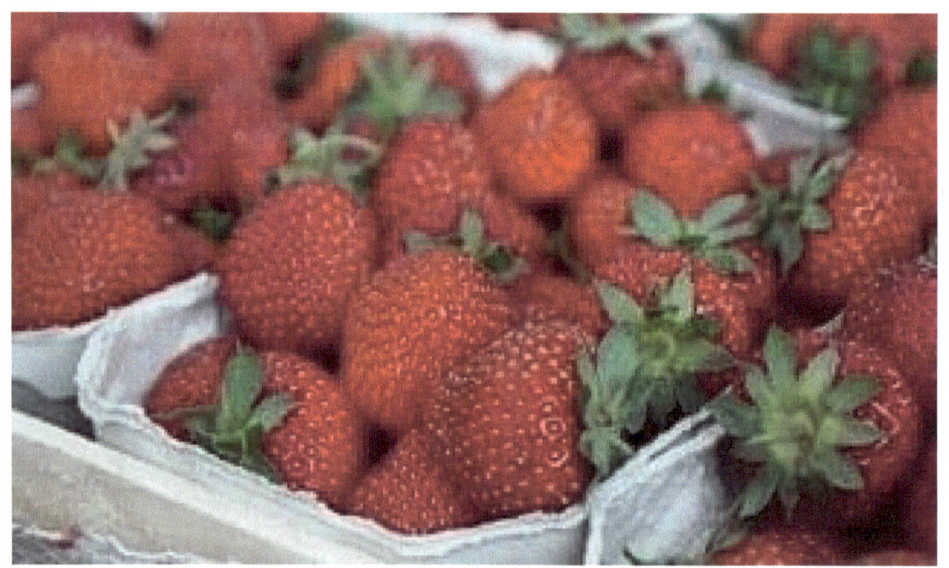

Nutrition Tips for Smoothie

Bananas
Mangoes
Apples
Clementines
Raspberries
Coconuts

Bananas

Bananas are an excellent source of vitamins, minerals, and fiber. They are full of potassium, which is an essential mineral that aids in cardiovascular health and helps maintain normal blood pressure levels. Bananas contain nutrients that moderate blood sugar levels as well as aid in digestion.

Mangoes

Mangoes are a super food that contain over 20 different vitamins and minerals. They are known to keep blood pressure under control, promote brain health, help clear acne, boost immunity, help manage and prevent diabetes, improve eye health and digestion, lower cholesterol, and alkalize the body.

Apples

An apple a day keeps the doctor away! Apples are one of the healthiest foods, full of phytonutrients, and antioxidants. They are very rich in fiber, which can help lower blood sugar and improve the digestive system. They are also high in vitamin C, which is an essential nutrient that has numerous important functions. Studies show that the components of an apple are important for optimal growth and overall wellness.

Clementines

Clementines are rich in a variety of nutrients such as calcium, magnesium, potassium, and phosphorus. They are also extremely high in vitamin C, which is an essential vitamin. Clementines are shown to be great for healthy skin, your immune system, strong bones and muscles, digestive health, cardiovascular health, electrolyte balance, and may even prevent cancer.

Raspberries

Raspberries are full of vitamins, minerals, and antioxidants that are extremely beneficial for your health. They are rich in phytonutrients, fiber, iron, magnesium, potassium, zinc, and much more. Raspberries are good for heart health, brainpower, cancer prevention, diabetes management, digestion and detox, increased immunity, and controlling inflammation.

Coconuts

There are numerous health benefits of coconuts. Eating a medium sized coconut will give you almost all of your daily-required vitamins and minerals. Coconuts are a saturated fat. They contain lauric acid, which increases HDL (good cholesterol) levels in the blood. Coconuts are high in dietary fiber, have a low glycemic index, improve digestion, and improve heart health.

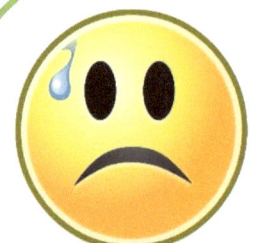

Lesson Plan 6: How to De-stress

Objectives:
- Learn what stress is and understand effects of stress
- Learn how to manage stress
- Learn what to eat and what not to eat to help prevent stress

Materials: Flip-chart sheets (plan for the day, keywords, recipe, attendance sheet), whiteboard, dry erase markers and eraser, name tags, 2 extension cords and extension strip, 2 kitchen knives, 4 cutting boards, 2 blenders, extension cord and power strip, tablecloth, 1 bowl and spoon per child, gloves, 30 medjool dates, date soaking water, 12 avocados, 12 teaspoons coconut oil, 12 tablespoons carob powder, 2 bananas

Plan for the Day

1. Exercise: Red Light, Green Light
Establish a starting line and finish line. Everyone begins along the starting line with one person calling out the lights. When you say "green light," all players will move as quickly as they can towards the finish line. When you say "red light," everyone must immediately stop moving. Players who keep moving when it is a red light are out. Start a new round when everyone gets across the finish line or when most players make it across the finish line.

2. Mindfulness
Get ready to relax. You can sit in a chair or lie down. Close your eyes and take a deep breath in. Now breathe out. Breathe in, and breathe out. Keep breathing slowly like this. Feel how it relaxes you to breathe deeply. One way to relax your body is by breathing deeply. Imagine that your body is like a balloon. When you breathe in, feel your chest and sides expanding, like a balloon filling with air. When you breathe out, imagine your body is like a balloon shrinking with the air being let out. Breathe in like a balloon being blown up. Now breathe out, like a balloon being emptied. Let the air out by blowing the air through your mouth. Keep breathing and simply relax. There is nothing you need to do right now except relax quietly. Be still for a moment, then open your eyes to look around the room. When you are ready, get up and return to your usual activities, feeling awake, but still feeling relaxed and calm.

Tell the children that visualization relaxation is a skill that can be learned; the more you practice, the more skilled you will become, and the more effectively you will be able to relax using visualization.

3. Ask the kids: What is stress?

- Act out an example of stress: One teacher will sit and pretend to do their homework at a table. Each teacher will then come up while teacher #1 is trying to concentrate. They will make noise, move around, ask him/her questions, try to clean the table teacher #1 is sitting at, etc.
- Break kids into groups of 4 with a teacher in each group. Help them to brainstorm 5 stressful situations and write them on the whiteboard. Have each group choose a stressful scenario without telling the other groups.
- Each group will then have 5 minutes to put together a quick skit to act their scenario out. One group acts out their stressful situation while the others sit as an audience and guess which scenario they are acting out.

4. Ask the kids: How do you de-stress? What helps you de-stress?
Go over the strategies to combat stress in children.
- Eat healthy, real foods
- Meditate (can use as an activity if time allows)
- Exercise
- Talk it out
- Sleep—how much sleep?

5. Recipe: Carob Mousse and Banana (see page 38)

6. Reflection: Share what they learned without repeating what others say.

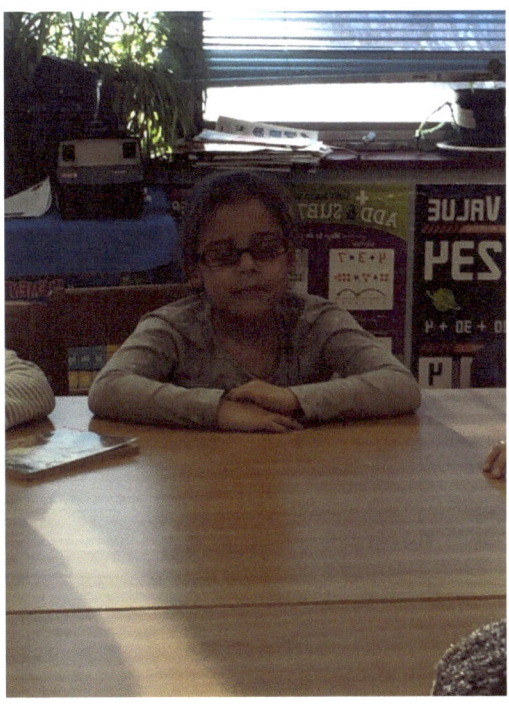

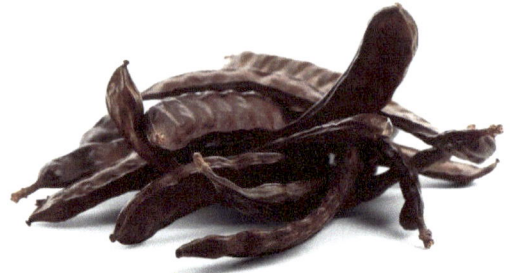

Carob Mousse and Banana
Servings: 3

Equipment
Blender
Kitchen knife
Measuring spoons

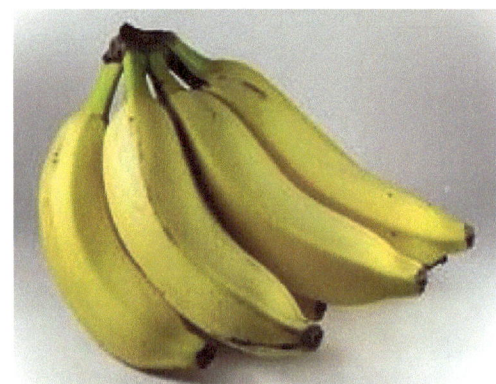

Ingredients
5 medjool dates, pitted and soaked in water
2 avocados
2 teaspoons coconut oil
2 tablespoons carob powder
2 bananas
¼-½ cup date soaking water as needed

Directions
1. Blend avocados, dates, coconut oil, and carob powder in a blender.
2. Thin mixture with soaking water from dates to desired consistency.
3. Serve with sliced banana or berries of your choice.
4. Enjoy right away or refrigerate.

Nutrition Tips for Carob Mousse and Banana

Medjool Dates
Avocados
Coconut Oil
Carob Powder

Medjool Dates

Dates are an energy-dense fruit that have a high content of natural glucose and fructose. Like apples, they are an excellent source of dietary fiber, which has numerous health benefits. Dates are also rich in potassium, which helps regulate blood pH levels and maintain intracellular fluid balance.

Avocados

Avocados are high in healthy fats. They also have an abundance of nutrients including vitamin K, folate, vitamin C, and potassium—more potassium than bananas! They are loaded with fiber and antioxidants. Avocados are known to help lower cholesterol and triglyceride levels, aid in losing weight, and may help prevent cancer.

Coconut Oil

Coconut oil has an abundance of health benefits. It helps prevent degenerative diseases, aids in weight loss, strengthens immunity, improves digestion system, protects against infections, and much more. It is also a good substitute for butter while cooking or baking!

Carob Powder

Carob is a type of shrub in the same family as peas. Due to its high vitamin and mineral content, it has a variety of health benefits including reducing the risk of cancer, improving digestion, boosting the immune system, preventing and managing diabetes, and preventing cardiovascular diseases.

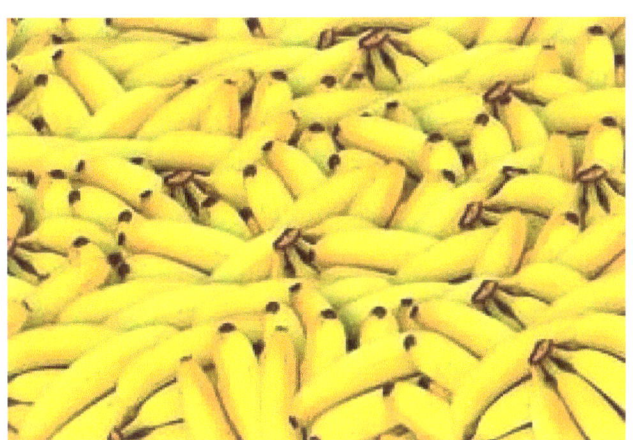

De-stress
Teacher Tips

What can stress do to us?
- Stress hurts our brain. Stress makes us:
  - Forget things and lose track of our thoughts
  - Have trouble in school
  - Worry a lot when there is nothing to worry about
  - Prone to bad moods and sometimes makes us sad or angry
  - Eat too much or too little

- Stress hurts our body. Stress can:
  - Give us a headache, chest pain, and a faster heartbeat
  - Make us dizzy and nauseous

How do we do to manage stress?
- Breathe deeply and purposefully (smell it, then cool it)
- Exercise to:
  - Release energy
  - Improve our ability to sleep
  - Increase our serotonin levels
- Eat nutritious food
- Think about something happy, something good that happened to us

We can also:
- Meditate
- Talk it out (share feelings with a friend)
- Sleep—how much sleep?
  - Ages 3-6 years need 10-12 hours a day
  - Ages 7-12 years need 10-11 hours a day
  - Ages 12-18 years need 8-9 hours a day

Foods that help us de-stress:
- **Avocados** help decrease blood pressure.
- **Apples** help our cells regenerate when stress threatens their lives.
- **Bananas** help to fight sleepiness and low blood sugar with carbohydrates.
- **Sweet potatoes** help boost our immune system and keep us strong.
- **Green vegetables** soothe the nerves and alleviate stress.
- **Nuts** lower blood pressure, give us healthy fats, and boost our immune system with vitamins and minerals.

Recap: <u>BEET</u> to de-stress
- **B**reathe
- **E**at well
- **E**xercise
- **T**hink about something that makes you happy

Let's De-stress!
Family Tip Sheet

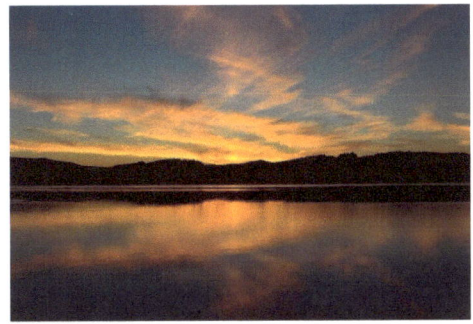

How does stress affect us?
- Everybody experiences stress in different ways.
- Stress targets the weakest part of our physiology or character.
- Normally stress can change a person in several different ways: emotionally, physically, behaviorally, or a combination of all three.
- Stress isn't avoidable, but it is manageable.

How to manage stress
- Breathe deeply and purposefully
- Exercise
- Eat nutritious food
- Think about something happy, something good that happened to us
- Keep a positive & realistic attitude
- Meditate

Foods that can help us de-stress
- Avocados help decrease blood pressure.
- Apples help our cells regenerate when stress threatens their lives.
- Bananas help to fight sleepiness and low blood sugar with carbohydrates.
- Sweet potatoes help boost our immune system and keep us strong.
- Green vegetables soothe the nerves and alleviate stress.
- Nuts lower blood pressure, give us healthy fats, and boost our immune system with vitamins and minerals.

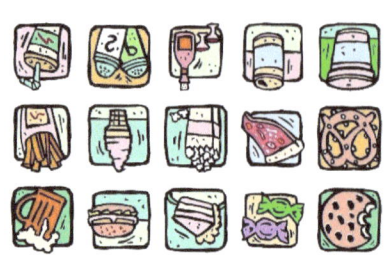

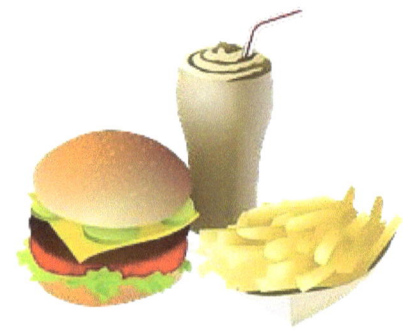

Lesson Plan 7: Good, Bad, and Ugly Fat

Objectives:
- Learn about fats, arteries, and cholesterol
- Learn how to properly support a healthy heart through nutrition

Materials: Flip-chart sheets (plan for the day, keywords, recipe, attendance sheet), whiteboard, dry erase markers and eraser, name tags, 2 extension cords and power strip, 2 kitchen knives, 2 spatulas, 4 cutting boards, 2 sets of measuring cups and spoons, food processor, 1 blender, tablecloth, 2 serving paper plates, gloves, 1 quart of filtered water, 1 mixing bowl, 3 head cauliflower, ground turmeric, dried mustard, 3 heads romaine lettuce, Himalayan salt, 6 dill pickles, 6 stalks of celery, 1 cup cashews soaked for 4 hours, 3 lemons, paprika

Plan for the Day

1. Exercise: Avoid the Octopus
Don't let the hungry octopus get you! First, pick one person to be the octopus. Then, draw two lines that are at least 20 feet apart. The other players, the fish, then line up on either line. When the octopus shouts "I'm hungry!" everyone tries to cross to the other side while the octopus tries to tag them. When a fish is tagged, he becomes a tentacle and must hold hands with the octopus, working with him to try to tag the other fish. The last fish left wins!

2. Mindfulness
To begin, make yourself comfortable. Adjust your clothing as needed and assume a comfortable position. Feel your body begin to relax. As your shoulders drop a little lower, your jaw loosens so your teeth are not touching, and your eyelids start to feel heavy. Take a deep breath in. Hold it, then slowly breathe out. Create a picture in your mind of the color red. Imagine red of all shades. You might picture red objects, a red landscape, or just a solid color. Imagine all the different tones of red. See roses, bricks, apples, and sunsets. Enjoy the color red. Now allow the color you are imagining to change to orange. Picture the color orange, infinite shades of orange, flowers, pumpkins, and carrots. Fill the entire visual field of your mind's eye with the color orange. Enjoy the color orange. Allow your attention to return to your breathing and notice how calm and regular your breathing is now.

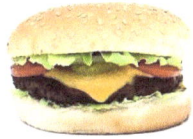

3. Activity: What are good fats and bad fats?

- What is fat? What happens to cooking fat when it cools? What happens to popcorn butter when you eat it?
    - Good fats/cholesterol: avocados, olives, coconuts, raw nuts
    - Bad fats/cholesterol: cake, cookies, French fries, bacon

- Tell the story of a man going for open-heart surgery. Ask the kids:
    - What do you think he had been eating on the way to the hospital emergency room?
    - What do you think his blood looked like?
    - Show test tube kit after the story.

- What did the doctors see when they opened the arteries? What are veins and arteries and their functions? Show clogged artery model to the children and explain what cholesterol does in the body.
    - Cholesterol floats around in your blood and can get into the walls of the blood vessels and stay there.
    - Too much cholesterol in the bloodstream can collect in the blood vessel walls, causing these "pipes" to become narrower.
    - Having too much cholesterol can clog the blood vessels and keep blood from moving freely the way it's supposed to. If the clogging gets worse over many years, it can cause damage to important body parts.

4. Recipe: Eggless "Egg" Salad Sandwich (see pages 44-45)

5. Reflection: Share what they learned without repeating what others say.

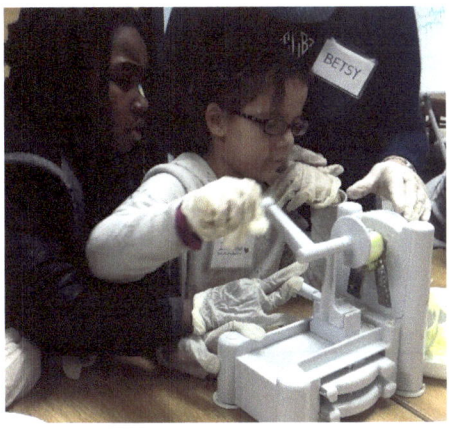

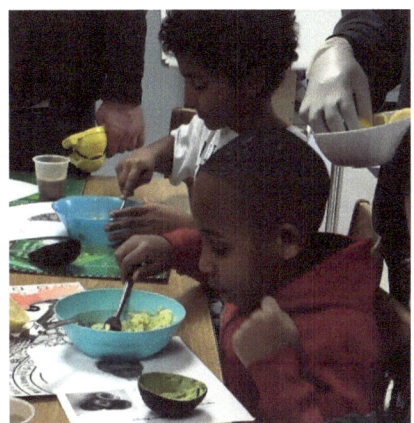

Eggless "Egg" Salad Sandwiches
*Recipe inspired by Aimee Perrin
Servings: 6

Equipment
Food processor
1 quart mixing bowl
Cutting board
Kitchen knife
Spatula
Measuring cups
Measuring spoons
Serving plates
Serving platter

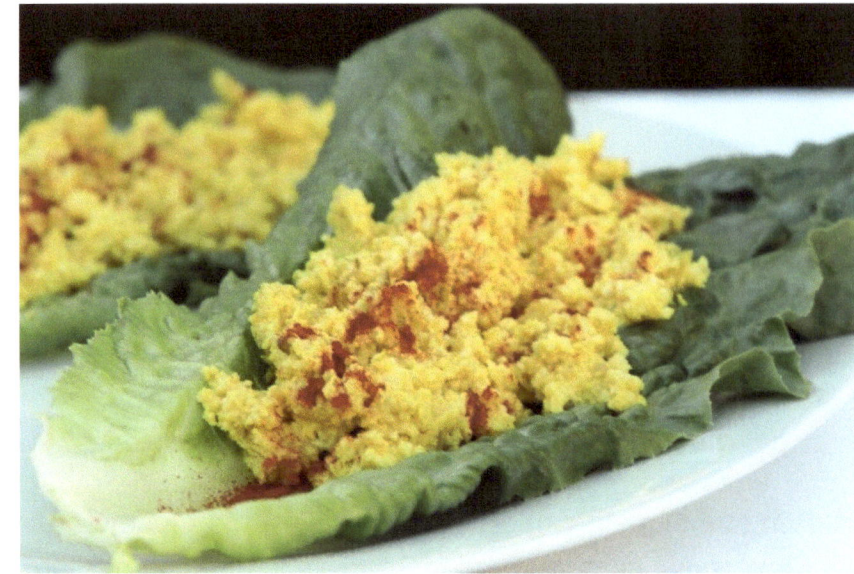

Salad Ingredients
1 head cauliflower
2 stalks celery
2 dill pickles (recommend the Real Pickles brand found in the refrigerated section of your health food store)

Mayo Ingredients
1 cup cashews, soaked at least 2 hours and drained well
2 tablespoons lemon juice
1/4 cup of filtered or spring water
1 1/2 teaspoon Celtic or Himalayan salt
1 teaspoon dry mustard
1 teaspoon turmeric
1 head of romaine lettuce

Directions

1. Remove leaves from cauliflower. Cut the head of the cauliflower into quarters and core each section. Break the cauliflower into pieces.

2. Place cauliflower into food processor and pulse until it's the size of rice. If you do not have a food processor, break up florets into rice sized pieces.

3. Place riced cauliflower into a large mixing bowl.

4. Chop celery and pickles into quarter inch cubes and add to mixing bowl.

5. Add mayo ingredients in the blender and cream it to the consistency of mayonnaise. Add a tablespoon at a time of water if too thick.

6. Add mayo to the cauliflower mixture and stir.

7. Chop off the end of the bunch of romaine lettuce. Wash well and either spin dry with a salad spinner or dry with paper towels.

8. Use only the medium-sized romaine leaves for the sandwiches.

9. Add a couple of tablespoons into a romaine leaf, sprinkle with a little paprika and roll up into a sandwich.

10. Serve and enjoy!

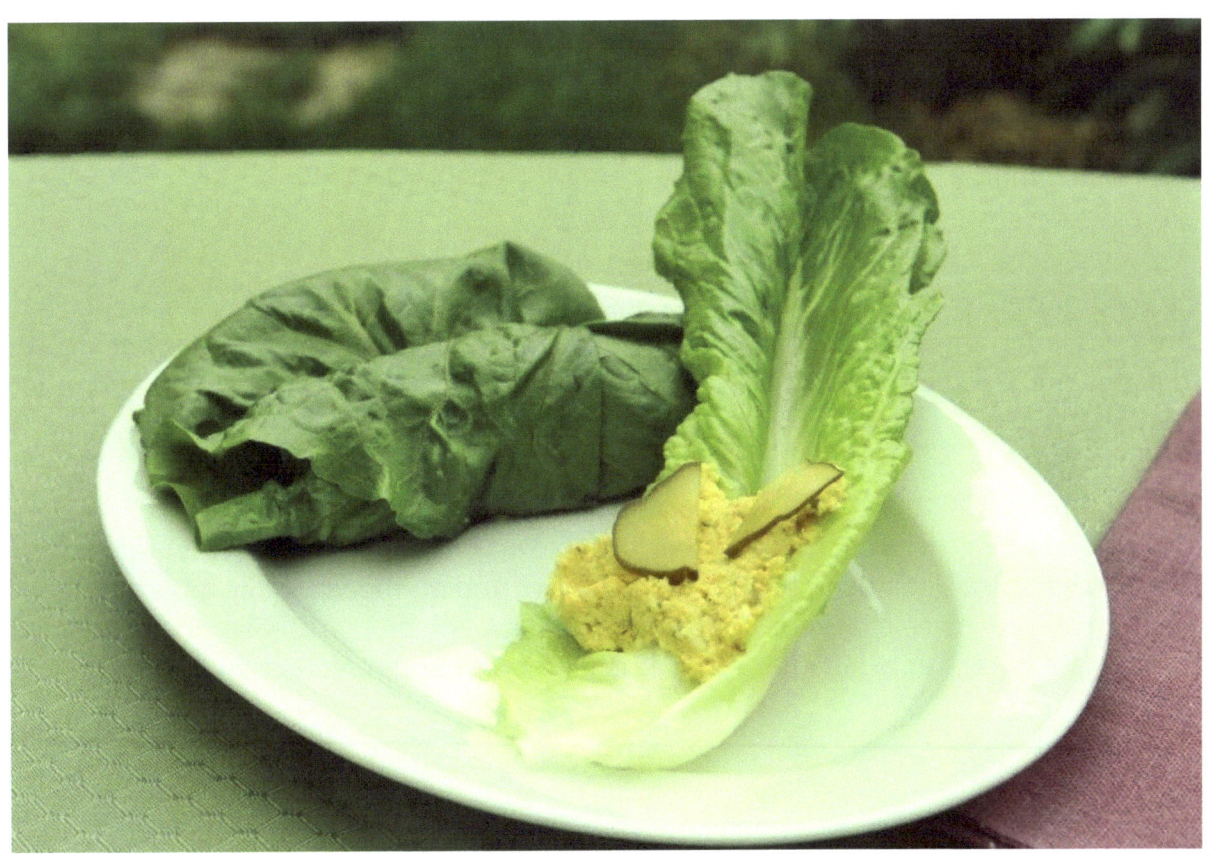

Nutrition Tips for Eggless "Egg" Salad Sandwiches
Cauliflower, Celery, Dill Pickles, Cashews, Lemon Juice, Dry Mustard, Turmeric

Cauliflower

Cauliflower has multiple fantastic health benefits. It is a great source of vitamin C, vitamin K, and folate. Cauliflower is an anti-inflammatory, aids in digestion, supports our cardiovascular system, and much more. Try sautéing it for a delicious and healthy side dish!

Celery

Celery is mostly made up of water, which means it is very low in calories. However, it still contains nutrients including vitamins K, C, A, and B. Unlike some vegetables, celery retains almost all of its nutrients even when cooked, so try steaming it!

Dill Pickles

If you didn't know, pickles are made from cucumbers! They are low in calories and contain some useful nutrients including calcium, potassium, phosphorus, and magnesium. They are also a good source of dietary fiber.

Cashews

Cashews are packed with fiber, vitamins, minerals, and phytochemicals that have numerous health benefits. They are high in monounsaturated fats that help lower bad LDL cholesterol and raise good HDL cholesterol. Cashews are full of potassium, iron, magnesium, and zinc.

Lemon Juice

Not only are lemons a super food, but they can also do wonders for any recipe and add so much flavor! The flavonoids in the juice are full of antioxidants. Lemon juice can soothe a sore throat, aid in digestion, support weight loss, bring down a fever, balance out pH levels, and much more.

Dry Mustard

Dry mustard powder comes from mustard seeds, which have several nutritional benefits. They contain a large amount of phytonutrients, which protect us from bacteria and viruses. Mustard seeds are also high in a variety of minerals including iron, magnesium, zinc, and calcium.

Turmeric

Turmeric is a spice that derives from the root of the *Curcuma longa* plant. It is a deep yellow-orange color that has been used in Chinese and Indian medicine for generations. Turmeric is known to lower cholesterol, protect against Alzheimer's disease, improve liver function, and is a potent anti-inflammatory. It is also an excellent source of iron and manganese.

Good, Bad, and Ugly Fats
Teacher Tips

What are the main types of fats?
- Saturated fats and trans fats – these are unhealthy fats that block your arteries, meaning the oxygen in the blood cannot get to your body. This can lead to heart disease and stroke.
    - Examples: beef, pork, chicken, sausages, bacon, and other meats from animals, eggs, dairy products, cream, butter, and processed foods including pies, donuts, and cakes
- Polyunsaturated fats and monounsaturated fats – these fats are good for health. They reduce the risk of heart disease and strokes by lowering bad cholesterol in your blood.
    - Examples: avocados, olives, nuts, and seeds

Tips to cut out bad fats:
- Use guacamole or hummus instead of butter or mayonnaise
- Limit your fast foods (pizzas, hamburgers, hot dogs, etc.)
- Eat vegetables, nuts, almond butter

What is cholesterol?
- Cholesterol is a type of fat found in your blood.
- You need cholesterol to help your brain, skin, and other organs grow and work the way they should.
- Too much cholesterol in the blood can clog the arteries that carry blood around your body.

What are the functions of veins and arteries?
- Your body has a highway system all its own that sends blood to and from your body parts. It's called the circulatory system and the roads are called arteries and veins.
    - **Arteries** carry bright red, oxygen-rich blood away from the heart to the rest of your body.
    - **Veins** return dark red deoxygenated blood back to the heart.

What happens to us when we eat bad fatty foods?
- If you have too much cholesterol in your bloodstream, it can collect in the blood vessel walls causing these "pipes" to become narrower.
- This can clog the blood vessels and keep blood from moving freely the way it's supposed to.
- If the clogging gets worse over many years, it can cause damage to important body parts like the heart (heart attack) and brain (stroke).
- Both kids and adults can have too much cholesterol in their blood.

Good, Bad, and Ugly Fats
Family Tip Sheet

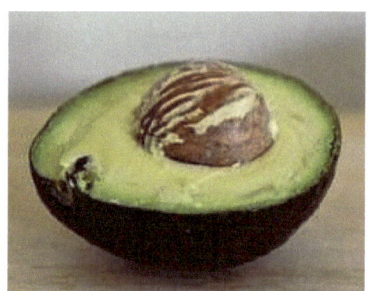

What's the difference between good fats and bad fats?

- Trans fats and saturated fats are bad fats. They will raise LDL (bad cholesterol) and lower HDL (good cholesterol). The reason that these fats are unhealthy is because they go through a process called hydrogenation, a chemical process that food manufacturers use to keep fat in packaged food from rotting.
- Mono- and polyunsaturated fats are good fats. Our body needs these good fats in order to get the essential vitamins A, D, E, and K. They promote cell development and are required to maintain a healthy immune system. These fats take a longer time to digest in the body, therefore keeping you fuller longer.

Examples of good and bad fats

Bad fats: butter, whole milk, sour cream, ice cream, bacon, fried foods, commercial baked goods, and fatty cuts of beef or pork

Good fats: nuts (almonds, cashews, walnuts), nut butters, olives, avocado, tofu, soybeans, and olive oil

Swapping bad fats for healthy fats

- Instead of using butter or margarine, use nut butters, avocado, or hummus
- Instead of having whole milk or whole milk yogurt, have coconut yogurt and almond, hemp, or coconut milk
- Instead of having ice cream for dessert, have some fruit with coconut yogurt

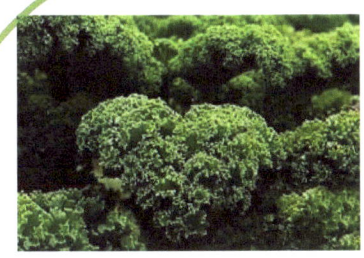

Lesson Plan 8:
Fabulous Fiber

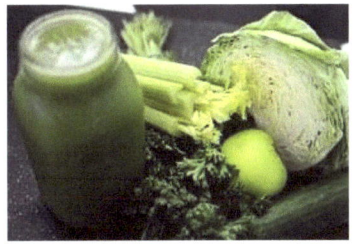

Objectives:

- Learn the importance of fiber
- Learn the amount of fiber in foods and how much fiber should be eaten daily
- Learn to make a meal plan for the correct amount of daily fiber

Materials: Flip-chart sheets (plan for the day, keywords, recipe, attendance sheet), whiteboard, dry erase markers and eraser, name tags, 2 extension cords and power strip, dehydrator, 2 kitchen knives, 4 cutting boards, 2 sets of cups, plastic knives, 2 blenders, very large mixing bowl, measuring cups, measuring spoons, lemon juicer, 20 paper plates, gloves, tablecloth, 2 bunches of curly kale, 1 bunch of red swiss chard, nutritional yeast, 3 lemons, 2 ½ cups of cashews, sea salt, 1 quart of water, pre-made kale chips

Plan for the Day

1. Exercise: I Am
Write the names of vegetables and fruits from all the lessons on slips of paper. Tape a slip of paper with the name of a vegetable or fruit to the back of each child without letting him or her know what it says. Children must then go around the room asking others yes or no questions to try and determine what they are. (e.g.: Am I red? Am I round? Do I grow on a tree?)

2. Mindfulness: Relax under pressure
Start by concentrating on your breathing. Breathe in and out. Deeply in and slowly out. Keep breathing slowly like this. You can slow your breathing even further by counting. Breathe in to the count of four, hold to the count of three, and breathe out to the count of five. Breathe in for four seconds, hold for three, exhale for five. Breathe in. Hold your breath. Breathe out. Breathe in and out again. You are learning the relaxation skill of slowing your breathing. You can feel yourself calming down as you breathe slowly and calmly. This calm breathing helps you to become focused, alert, and relaxed. You are learning how to relax under pressure. Continue to breathe slowly. Every so often just notice your breathing and focus on allowing your breathing to slow down.

3. Activity: Building a meal around fiber
- What is fiber?
- <u>Fiber</u>: Plant matter that cannot be broken down in the stomach.
  - Moves food through the digestive system
  - Show red swiss chard and identify the veins
  - Draw a picture of the veins on red swiss chard and the outline of the leaf.
  - Label the veins and label the picture "Fiber in red swiss chard"

- Why is fiber important?
  - Acts as a toothbrush and cleans plaque
  - Fiber helps move food through the digestive system.
  - Veins brings water, oxygen, and nutrients to the rest of the plant and support it
  - Review the life cycle of plants and how fiber is important and nourishes plants.

- Break into groups of two or three children. Using three paper plates and pictures of food with values of fiber in grams on them, create breakfast on one plate, lunch on a second, and supper on a third plate. Make sure the amount of fiber does not exceed 25 grams for the day. Photograph children with their meals.

4. What is in the bag?
- Put a bunch of curly green kale in a paper bag and get the children to guess what it is.
- Open the bag slightly and ask them to sniff its contents without looking or touching.
- Ask the children to describe what they can smell.
- Next, ask one or more children to feel the kale and describe it without looking.
- Finally, allow the children to see a little part of the vegetable and if they haven't done so already to tell you what they think it is.
- Reveal the kale. Tell the children that this is a very special vegetable and that they are going to be finding out lots of information about it.
- Ask the children if they have eaten kale and if so what they think of it.

5. Recipe: Cheezy Kale Chips (see page 51)

6. Reflections: Share what they learned without repeating what others say.

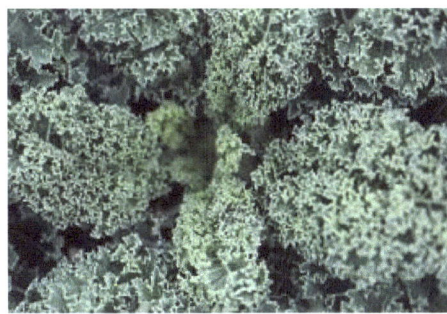

Cheezy
Kale Chips
Servings: 2

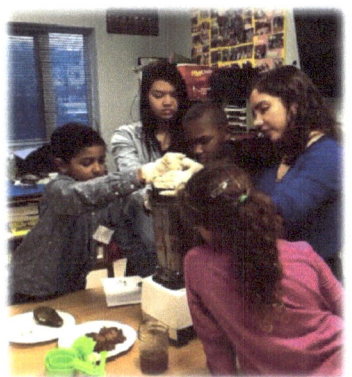

Equipment
Dehydrator
Large mixing bowl
Cutting board
Kitchen knife
Blender
Measuring cups
Measuring spoons

Ingredients
1 large bunch of curly green kale, washed, large stems removed, torn into bite size pieces

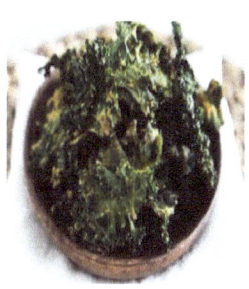

Coating
1 ¼ cup cashews, soaked 2 hours
3 tablespoons lemon juice
1 tablespoon nutritional yeast
1 teaspoon Himalayan pink crystal salt (use more or less to taste)

Directions
1. Put coating ingredients in the blender. Blend until smooth.
2. Using your hands, massage coating onto kale pieces, getting it inside the curls. Put on teflex sheets. Don't worry about flattening them—they're better bunched up.
3. Dehydrate at 105º F overnight or until coating is dry and kale is very crispy.

Nutrition Tips for Cheezy Kale Chips
Kale
Cashews
Lemon
Nutritional Yeast

Kale
Kale is one of the healthiest vegetables in the world. It has over 45 different flavonoids, which are powerful antioxidants that have a multitude of health benefits. Kale is an excellent source of vitamin C and is known to help lower cholesterol, prevent cancer, prevent and manage diabetes, and is good for brain and bone health.

Cashews
Cashews are packed with fiber, vitamins, minerals, and phytochemicals that have numerous health benefits. They are high in mono-unsaturated fats that help lower bad LDL cholesterol and raise good HDL cholesterol. Cashews are full of potassium, iron, magnesium, and zinc.

Lemon
The benefits of lemons are endless. Lemon juice is an excellent source of vitamin C, can help relieve indigestion and constipation, is used in skin care and weight loss, can be used to treat respiratory disorders and rheumatism, balance pH levels, and even flush out toxins.

Nutritional Yeast
Nutritional yeast is a dietary supplement often used by vegetarians that provides vitamin B-12. It is gluten free and is high in protein, fiber, and folic acid. You can add nutritional yeast to your diet in salads, smoothies, pasta, snack foods, and so much more!

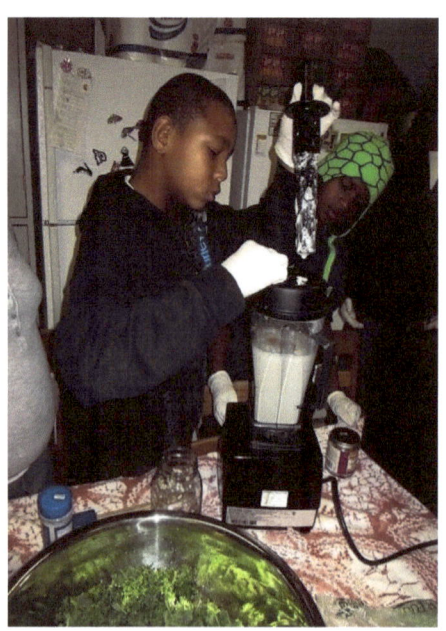

Fabulous Fiber
Teacher Tips

What is fiber?
- The term fiber refers to carbohydrates that cannot be digested. Fiber is found in the plants we eat for food—fruits, vegetables, grains, and legumes.

Types of fiber:
- Soluble fiber partially dissolves in water and has been shown to lower cholesterol.
- Insoluble fiber does not dissolve in water, which is why it helps with constipation.

Why is fiber important for us?
- Fiber plays an important role in supporting a healthy digestive system.
- It regulates bowel movements and may potentially reduce the risk of colon cancer.
- It helps keep the body's system clean and running smoothly.
- Foods that are high in fiber also have the benefit of being filling, which can help discourage overeating.
- When combined with ample fluid intake, fiber helps move food through the digestive system and might reduce the risk of certain cancers, diabetes, heart disease, and digestive disorders.

What happens when we do not have enough fiber?

- *Poor digestive health*—Diets low in fiber or high in fat increase the risk for constipation, diverticular disease, and hemorrhoids.
- *Cardiovascular disease*—Elevated levels of total and LDL cholesterol in the blood significantly increase the risk of arterial diseases, such as coronary heart disease and stroke. Lifestyle habits including consuming a low-fiber diet contribute to these higher cholesterol panels. Increased fiber intake has also been found to help reduce high blood pressure.
- *Weight gain*—When a diet consistently lacks high-fiber foods, weight gain is a risk. Fiber helps satisfy hunger and discourage overeating. High-fiber foods generally require more chewing time and are digested more slowly than refined carbohydrates or sugars, which helps keep the stomach feeling full longer.
- *Poor blood sugar control*—Low-fiber, refined carbohydrates, such as white bread and sugary foods, get digested quickly in the body, leading to a quicker rise in blood sugar. Research shows that dietary fiber in foods may reduce the risk of type 2 diabetes.

Good sources of fiber for kids
A high-fiber food has 5 grams or more of fiber per serving, and a good source of fiber is one that provides 3 grams per serving. Some of the best sources of fiber include:
- Grains: Whole grain breads and cereals, oat bran, brown rice, and barley
- Fruits: Apples, oranges, bananas, berries, prunes, and pears
- Vegetables: Green peas, artichokes, baked potatoes with skin, and legumes (e.g., dried beans, split peas, and lentils)

Fabulous Fiber
Family Tip Sheet

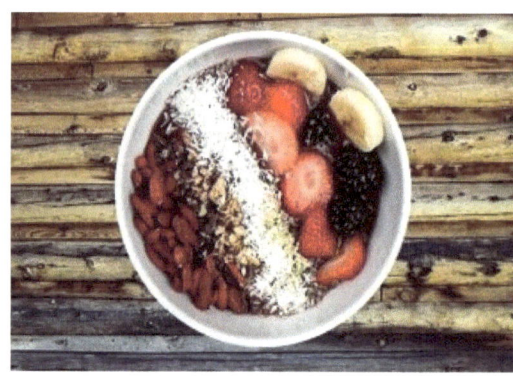

What is fiber?

- The term fiber refers to carbohydrates that cannot be digested. Fiber is found in plant foods—fruits, vegetables, grains, and legumes.
- There are two different types of fiber: soluble fiber and insoluble fiber.
  - Soluble fiber partially dissolves in water and has been shown to lower cholesterol.
  - Insoluble fiber does not dissolve in water and acts like a toothbrush cleaning the digestive tract. That's why it helps with constipation.

Why is fiber good for you?

Fiber plays an important role in supporting a healthy digestive system.

- It regulates bowel movements and may potentially reduce the risk of colon cancer.
- It helps keep the body's system clean and running smoothly.
- Foods that are high in fiber also have the benefit of being filling, which can help discourage overeating.
- When combined with ample fluid intake, fiber helps move food through the digestive system and might reduce the risk of certain cancers, diabetes, heart disease, and digestive disorders.

Where can you get fiber?

- Grains: Whole grain breads and cereals, oat bran, brown rice, and barley
- Fruits: Apples, oranges, bananas, berries, prunes, and pears
- Vegetables: Green peas, artichokes, baked potatoes with skin, and legumes (e.g., dried beans, split peas, and lentils)

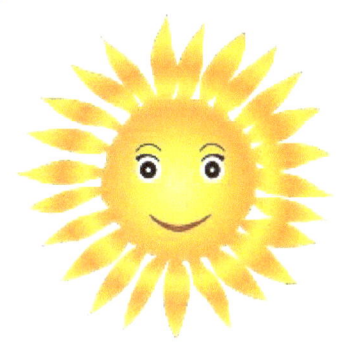

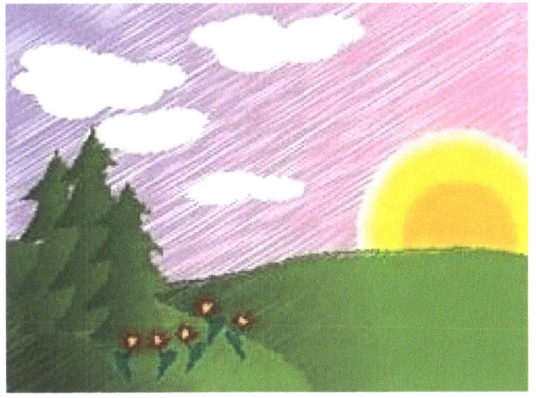

Lesson Plan 9: The Life Cycle of a Plant

Objectives:
- Understand connection between the sun and all living things
- Gain familiarity with the components of photosynthesis

Materials: Flip-chart sheets (plan for the day, keywords, recipe, attendance sheet), whiteboard, dry erase markers and eraser, name tags, *Living Sunlight* by Molly Bang, gloves, dehydrator, Spirooli, measuring spoon, paper plates, plastic knives, pre-made apple chips, 3 fuji apples, ground cinnamon

Plan for the Day

1. Exercise: Hula Hoop Relay Race
Divide group into two teams. The players on each team join hands to form a line. Loop a hula hoop over one player's arm. Without letting go of the other players' hands, he or she must step into and through the hoop so it rests on his or her other arm then slide it onto the next player's arm so he or she can repeat the same maneuver. Whichever team can pass the hoop to the front of the line and back first without letting go of each other's hands is the winner.

2. Mindfulness
Find a comfortable position. For the next few moments, calm your mind by focusing on your breathing. Allow you breathing to center and relax you. Breathe in and out. Now begin to create a picture in your mind of a place where you can completely relax. Imagine what this place needs to be like in order for you to feel calm and relaxed. Start with the physical layout of the place you are imagining. Where is this peaceful place? You might envision somewhere outdoors or indoors. It may be a small place or large one. Create an image of this place. Focus now on the sights of your place— colors, shapes, objects, plants, water, and all the beautiful things that make your place enjoyable. Picture yourself in your peaceful place. This moment you are imagining now, you can picture again the next time you need to relax.

3. Introduction: Keywords of the day and review

- New keywords
    - <u>Photosynthesis</u> – the cycle of plants and how they make energy. The plant absorbs all water, nutrients, and carbon dioxide and produces sugar and oxygen.
    - <u>Water</u> – molecules made of one part hydrogen and two parts oxygen; needed by plants for photosynthesis. Review water cycle.
    - <u>Carbon dioxide</u> – gas in the air needed by plants to "breathe" in order to photosynthesize. (What people breathe out and plants breathe in.)

4. Activity

- Read *Living Sunlight* book
- Living Sunlight (Photosynthesis) skits in groups
    - Divide children into groups of 4-5. In each group, one person is the seed, one person is the sun, one person waters the seed, and one person is the air. (Additional roles may be earthworm or animal.)
    - Allow 2-3 minutes to prepare skit.
    - Groups take turns acting out their skits for the audience.

5. Recipe: Cinnamon Apple Chips (see page 57)

6. Reflection: Share what they learned without repeating what others say.

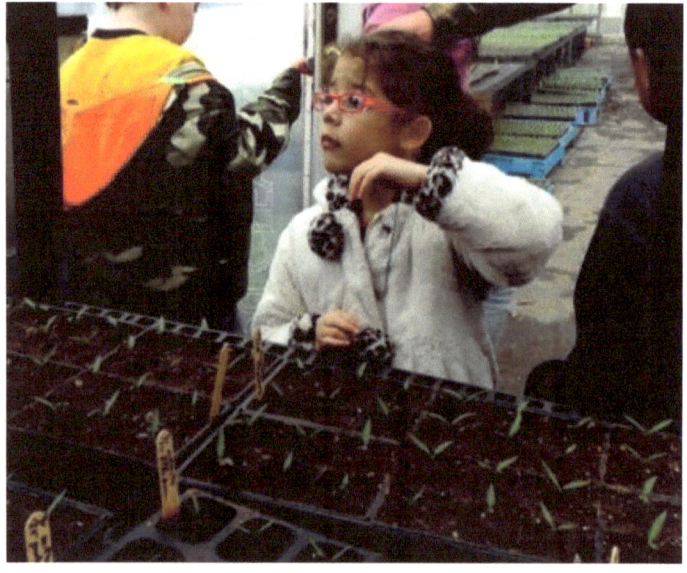
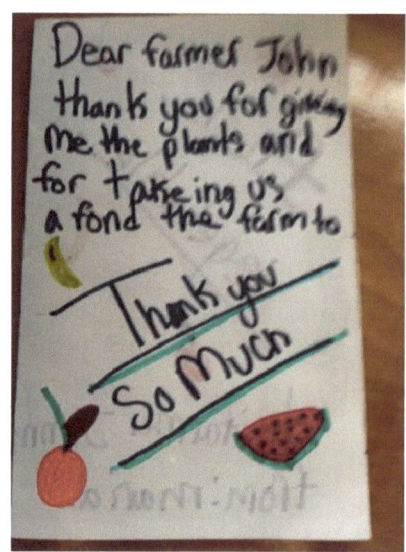

Cinnamon Apple Chips
Servings: 3

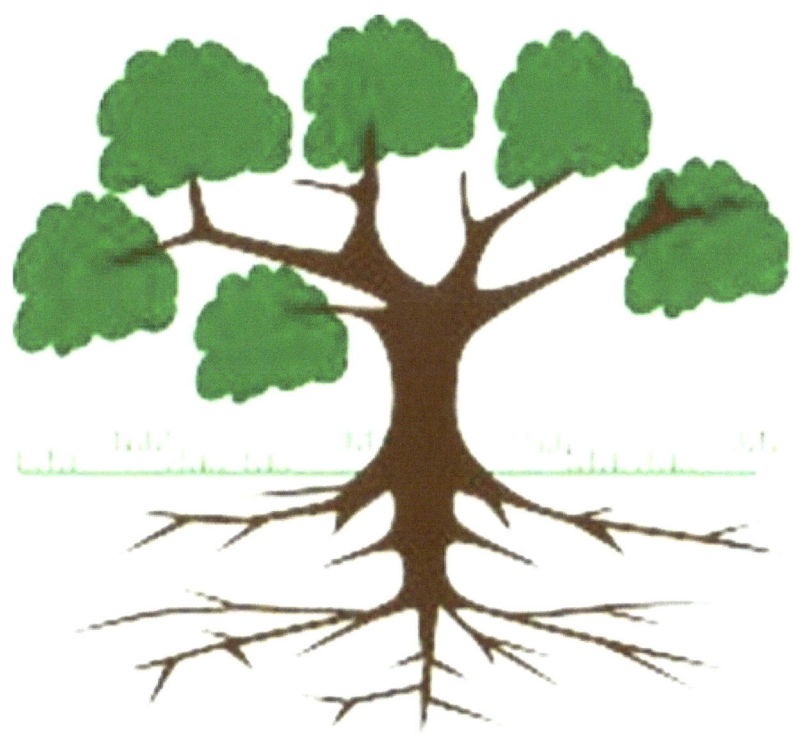

Equipment
Spirooli, mandolin, or knife
Dehydrator

Ingredients
3 to 4 ripe organic apples
1 tablespoon ground cinnamon
1 tablespoon granulated sweetener of your choice (optional)

Directions
1. Slice the tops off the apples. If desired, core and peel the apples. Next, slice into thin rounds, approximately 1/8" to 1/4" thick. A Spirooli or mandolin works best for uniform thickness. Remove the seeds if apples have not been cored.
2. Toss the sliced apples with cinnamon and sugar (optional) and arrange in a single layer in your dehydrator or on a parchment paper-lined baking pan.
3. Turn the dehydrator or oven to 115º F. Allow the apples to dehydrate for 6 to 8 hours or until they are dried and as crisp as you want them to be.

<u>Nutrition Tips for Apple Chips</u>
Apples
Cinnamon

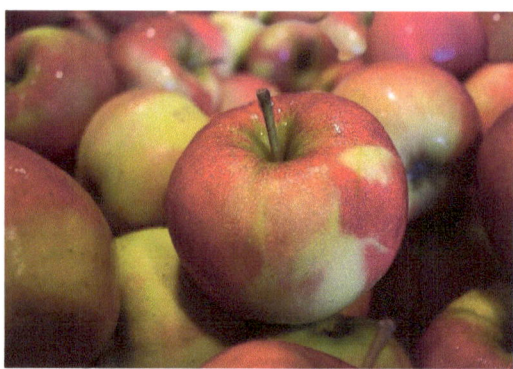

Apples

Apples are full of phytonutrients that can aid in regulating your blood sugar levels. Apples also have high amounts of fiber. Eating a diet high in fiber has many health benefits including reducing the risk of certain diseases, controlling blood sugar and blood fat levels, and maintaining your digestive tract.

Cinnamon

Cinnamon is a potent antioxidant that has various health benefits. It has anti-inflammatory compounds that can boost brain function, boost immunity, lower bad cholesterol, and regulate blood sugar.

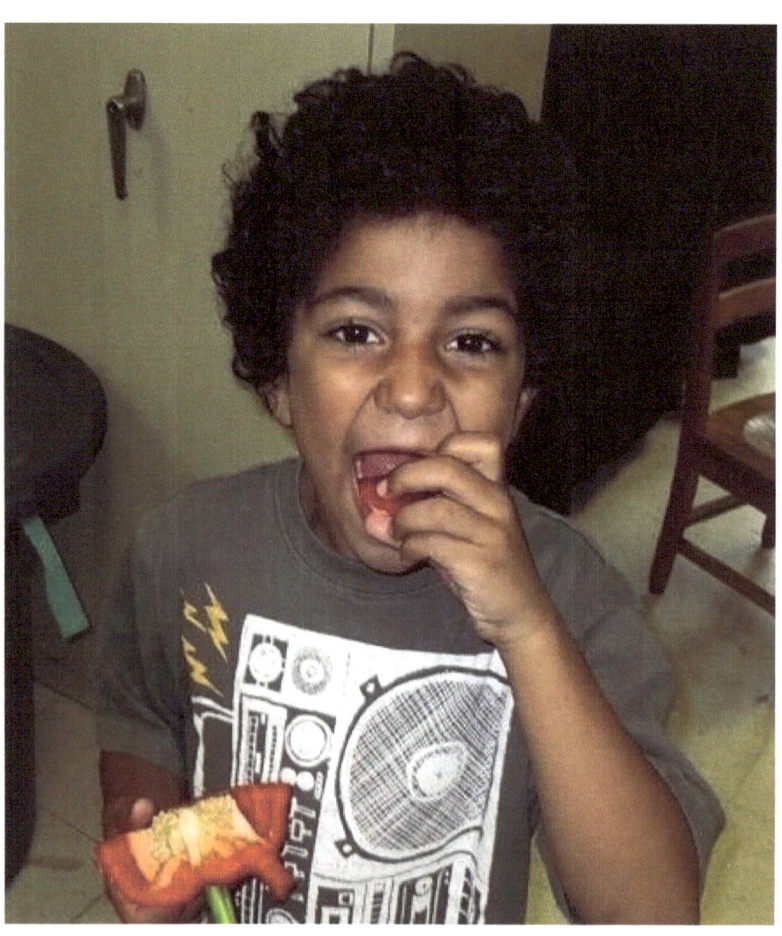

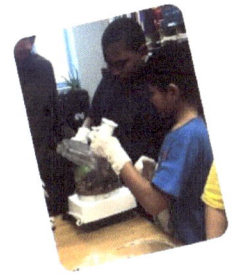

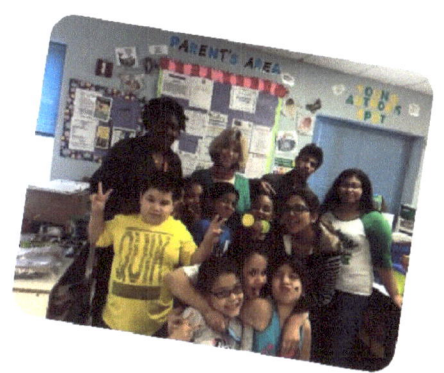

Lesson Plan 10:
Grand Finale

Objectives:
- Discover what we have learned
- Create a lasting memory—designing mugs
- Prepare Almond Butter Banana Ice Cream

Materials: Flip-chart sheets (plan for the day, keywords, recipe, attendance sheet), whiteboard, dry erase markers and eraser, name tags, 2 extension cords and extension strip, 2 kitchen knives, 4 cutting boards, mugs, plastic knives, 2 food processors, measuring spoons, 1 bowl and spoon per child, gloves, tablecloth, 20 bananas, organic natural almond butter, water

Plan for the Day

1. Exercise: Freeze Tag
Begin by choosing a person to be "it" who will freeze other players. When the game begins, everyone runs away from the person who is "it." The one who is "it" chases after other players, trying to tag (touch) them. If a person is successfully tagged, he or she must freeze in place (stand still and not move). Frozen people cannot move until another player un-freezes them by tagging them so they return to normal. The player who is "it" wins by freezing all players.

2. Mindfulness: Floating on a cloud
First, relax your body. Starting at the top of your head, allow a feeling of relaxation to begin. Feel the relaxation grow with each breath you take. Breathe in, feeling the relaxation continuing to your arms and hands. Breathe out the tension. Breathe in relaxation. Allow your chest and upper back to relax and release the tension as you exhale. Continue to breathe in relaxation and breathe out tension. Now you are feeling deeply relaxed. Begin to create a picture in your mind. Imagine that you are floating on a soft, fluffy white cloud. Feel the surface beneath you becoming softer, more cloudlike. Feel the clouds rising out of the surface you are on, surrounding you in protective support. Soon you are floating on just the cloud. Let it rise a little further, taking you with it. See the walls and ceiling around you disappearing as you float into the sunny sky, drifting on the cloud.

3. Jeopardy Review: What we learned in 10 weeks

4. Recipe: Almond Butter Banana Ice Cream (see page 61)

5. Reflections: Share what they learned without repeating what others say.

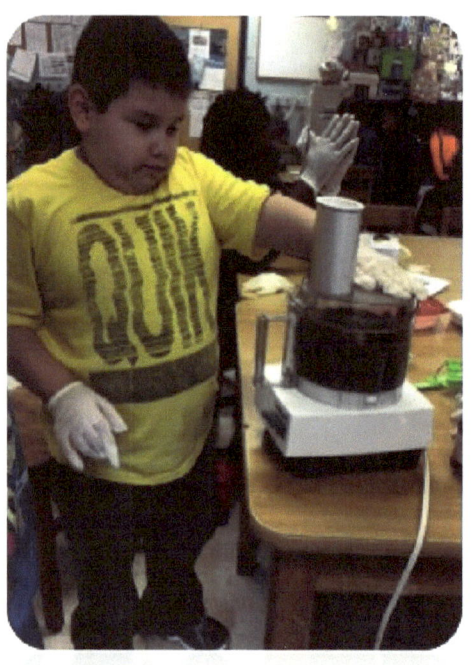 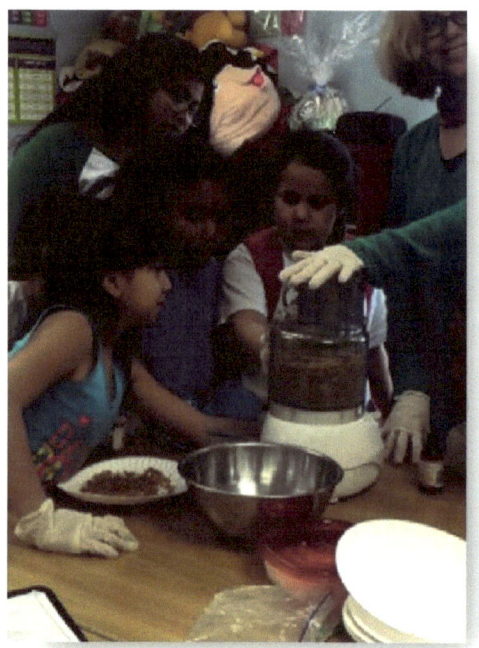

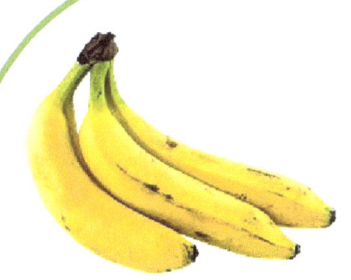
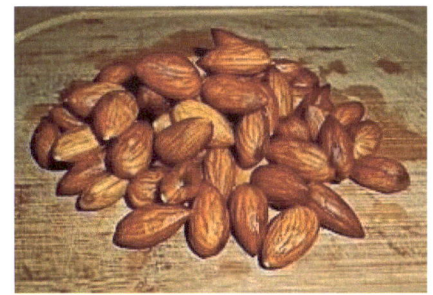

Almond Butter Banana Ice Cream
Servings: 2

Equipment
Food Processor

Ingredients
2 frozen bananas
2 tablespoons organic natural almond butter
Water if needed to facilitate blending

Directions
1. Break the frozen bananas into chunks and toss them into a mini food processor along with the almond butter. Add a pinch of Himalayan sea salt if using unsalted almond butter (optional).

2. Blend until the bananas break down into a soft-serve consistency, adding a tablespoon or two of water to help facilitate blending if necessary. The result should be a creamy, uniform ice cream.

3. Serve immediately for a soft-serve style dessert, or transfer to a sealed container and store in the freezer for a firmer, scoop-able ice cream.

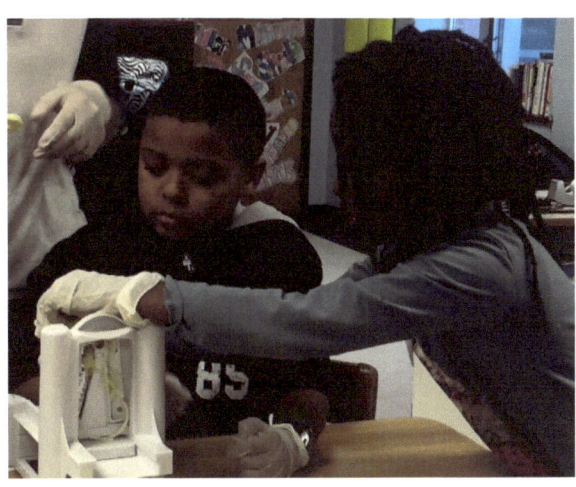
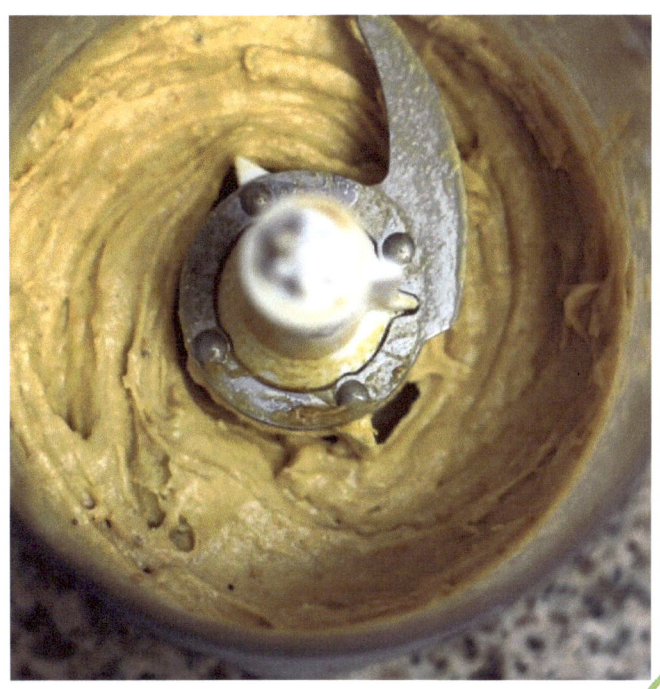

Nutrition Tips for Almond Butter Banana Ice Cream
Bananas
Almond Butter

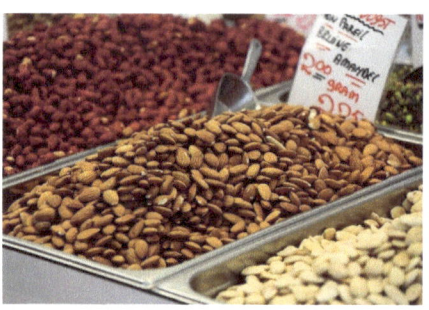

Bananas

Bananas are an excellent source of vitamins, minerals, and fiber. They are full of potassium, which is an essential mineral that aids in cardiovascular health and helps maintain normal blood pressure levels. Bananas contain nutrients that moderate blood sugar levels as well as aid in digestion.

Almond Butter

Almond butter contains healthy monounsaturated fat that is necessary for our bodies. Almond butter is full of magnesium, which is good for heart health. It is also rich in potassium, which is essential for maintaining blood pressure. You can use almond butter in a variety of recipes including smoothies, sandwiches, baked goods, and much more!

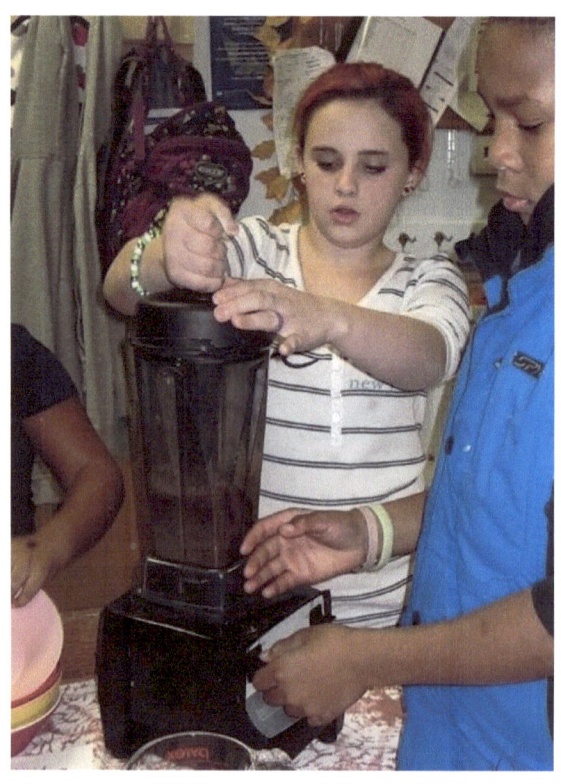

Appendix 1
RKRF Physical Activities

Ages 5 - 7 Outdoor Activities

- **Jump Rope Challenge**: Two people hold either end of the jump rope and swing the rope in the same direction. Children will try to jump in and over the rope, taking one or two jumps before safely exiting the swinging rope. When a child fails to join in, jump over, or exit the swinging rope (interrupting the swings), he or she is out until the next round.

- **Avoid the Octopus**: Don't let the hungry octopus get you! First, pick one person to be the octopus. Then, draw two lines that are at least 20 feet apart. The other players, the fish, then line up on either line. When the octopus shouts "I'm hungry!" everyone tries to cross to the other side while the octopus tries to tag them. When a fish is tagged, he becomes a tentacle and must hold hands with the octopus, working with him to try to tag the other fish. The last fish left wins!

- **Banana Relay Race:** Children will be split up into teams for the relay race with a banana used as the baton. After the race, explain why bananas are good to eat after exercising. (They contain protein and good carbs to help with muscle recovery and potassium prevents muscle cramping.)

- **Turkey Trot**: Arrange the kids into several groups and give each group a Thanksgiving name (Mayflower, Plymouth Rock, Turkeys, Pilgrims, etc.). Choose one group to be a tagger in the center and position the other groups on opposite sides. When one of the groups is called to run, they have to get to the opposite side without being tagged by the center group. If tagged, they must go back to their starting line. After all the groups have been called, have a new group to be the tagger and all the groups will return to their starting position.

Ages 5 - 7 Inside Activities

- **Musical Chairs**: Make a circle of chairs with one less chair than the total number of children. Staff uses a list of questions related to the lesson. Using "fruits and vegetables" songs, play the music for a few seconds while the children circle the chairs. When the music stops, the child without a chair is asked to answer a question. (See suggested questions below.) If the child does not answer it correctly, he or she may ask a friend for help answering it. If it still is not answered correctly, they both are out of the circle. If a correct answer is provided, begin the music again. For every child eliminated from the game, remove a chair from the circle.

- Suggested Questions for Musical Chairs
    - Name a yellow fruit.
    - Name a red fruit.
    - Name an orange fruit.
    - When you are thirsty, what is the best thing to drink?
    - Name a good fat.
    - Name a powerful vegetable protein.
    - What is fiber?
    - Name a big orange vegetable.
    - Name a green vegetable.
    - Name a red vegetable.
    - Name a healthy grain.
    - How much water should you drink a day?
    - What percent of your body is water?
    - What percent of mother Earth is water?
    - Name a vegetable with vitamin C.
    - Name a vegetable with vitamin E.

- **Duck, Duck, Goose:** In this game, kids sit down in a circle facing each other. One person is "it" and walks around the circle. As they walk around, they tap people's heads and say whether they are a "duck" or a "goose." Once someone is picked as the goose, they get up and try to chase "it" around the circle. The goal is to tap that person before they are able sit down in the goose's spot. If the goose is not able to do this, they become "it" for the next round and play continues. If they do tap the "it" person, the person tagged must sit in the center of the circle. Then the goose becomes "it" for the next round. The person in the middle can't leave until another person is tagged and they are replaced.

- **Hokey Pokey:** Invite children to sing and act out the song "Hokey Pokey." Before you begin, have the children feel the pulses in their necks. Have children stand in a circle and sing. Verses include putting in the left arm, right arm, left foot, right foot, both arms and whole self. When children have finished the song, have them feel the pulses in their necks again. Ask them what they notice about their pulses and help them conclude that their pulses got faster because their hearts were beating faster after they did physical activities. Ask children to name other activities that make their hearts work harder.

- **Keep Away**, also called Monkey in the Middle, is a children's game in which two or more players must pass a ball to one another while a player in the middle attempts to intercept it.

Ages 8 - 12 Indoor Activities

- **Simon Says:** This game is for three or more players. One player takes the role of "Simon" and issues instructions—usually physical actions such as "jump in the air" or "stick out your tongue"—to the other players. Instructions should only be followed if prefaced with the phrase "Simon says." For example: "Simon says touch your nose." If players make a mistake or follow instructions given without the phrase "Simon says," they are out.

- **Balloon Tag (also called Popper Stomper)**
Sent in by: Kelsey of Salt Lake City, UT

Ready, set... stomp and pop!
This is a game for 6 or more players and should be played outside or in an open area. To play, all you need are balloons and string. There aren't any teams in this game. It's every player for him or herself.
The object of the game is to pop the other players' balloons before they pop yours. Players run around and try to stomp other players' balloons while keeping other players from stomping on theirs. Last player left with their balloon wins. Start stomping!

- **Fruit Tag**
Sent in by: Elizabeth of Maynard, MA

Everyone chooses the name of a fruit and says it out loud. One person starts off being "it." "It" runs toward a player. That player has to call out another player's fruit before "it" has time to tag her. "It" then runs to the new player and tries to tag her before she yells out another player's fruit. If "it" tags someone before she yells out another player's fruit, she becomes "it."

- **I Woke Up Saturday Morning**
Sent in by: Cauley of SC

Don't be caught napping when the clapping starts! This is a clapping game.
Players sit in a circle and put both hands out in front of them with palms facing up. Overlap hands so your right hand is above the left hand of the person sitting on your right. (Get it?!) One person starts by reaching over with their right hand and clapping the right hand of the person sitting on their left.
The clap is passed around the circle while players count. If a player's hand is clapped on "three," that player is out. If the player pulls her hand away in time, and the person claps their own hand, then that person is out.

When there are only two people left in the game, the hand positions change. Player 1 holds both hands out, palms facing up.

Player 2 slaps player 1's hands with both of his hands, palms facing down. Now player 2 holds his hands out, and player 1 slaps his hands.

Play continues until there is only one person left!

- **Land, Sea, Air**

Sent in by: Natalie of Santa Clara, CA

This game is for 5 or more people and should be played outside or in an open area. To play this game, you just need to draw a line on the ground.

Pick one person to be the caller.

The caller calls out the commands **land**, **sea**, or **air**.

If the caller says **land**, everyone jumps behind the line. If the caller says **sea**, everyone jumps over the line.

If the caller says **air**, everyone jumps up.

If **land** or **sea** is called twice in a row, the second time, you don't move. If **air** is called twice in a row, jump up both times.

If you jump on the line or make a mistake, you're out.

The last person still jumping is the winner.

- **I Am**

Write the names of vegetables and fruits from all the lessons on slips of paper.

Tape a slip of paper with the name of a vegetable or fruit to the back of each child without letting him or her know what it says.

Children must then go around the room asking others yes or no questions to try and determine what they are. (e.g.: Am I red? Am I round? Do I grow on a tree?)

- **Hot Potato**

Queue up a song and have children stand in a circle. While music is playing, pass a fruit, vegetable, or processed food around the circle. When the music stops, the child holding the food must say a benefit of the natural product or say why the processed product is not good. The child has 10 seconds to answer or step out. Those who have stepped out can choose the product for the group. Try using the following: apple, banana, beet, carrot, avocado, celery, cucumber, orange, pear, nut, junk cereal, mac and cheese.

- **Steal the Bacon**

1. Children separate into two teams. They line up on each side facing each other.
2. Place an eraser on the stool in between the two teams
3. Each child is given a number in ascending order beginning at one on one side while each child is numbered in descending order on the opposing team. Children should never be facing their opponent who has the same number.
4. Staff member calls out a number and the children assigned to that number run to the stool. The first one to grab the eraser and run past their line gets a point.
5. The opponent can tag the child he's playing against and stop him from getting a point. If the child is tagged, neither team gets a point.
6. The eraser goes back on the stool and a new number is called.

- **Hula Hoop Relay Race**

Divide group into two teams. The players on each team join hands to form a line. Loop a hula hoop over one player's arm. Without letting go of the other players' hands, he or she must step into and through the hoop so it rests on his or her other arm then slide it onto the next player's arm so he or she can repeat the same maneuver. Whichever team can pass the hoop to the front of the line and back first without letting go of each other's hands is the winner.

Appendix 2
Presidential Fitness Program

Stretches for warm-up and cool-down

Neck stretch: Tilt head from resting position to the left or right until you feel resistance, then hold for 10-30 seconds. Return to resting position and repeat on other side.

Reach to the sky: Place feet shoulder width apart and raise both hands up with wrists crossed and palms grasping each other, then hold for 10-30 seconds.

Reach back: Place feet shoulder width apart with arms at your sides, then slowly move arms back with your thumbs facing down.

Arm circles: Place feet shoulder width apart with arms straight out to the side and palms facing up. Slowly move arms in small circles. As the warm-up continues begin making larger circles. Once the arm circles are as large as possible, stop and reverse.

Toe touch: Sit on a flat surface with your legs fully extended out in front of you. Extend arms out in front of you and reach out to touch your toes.

Twister: Sit on a flat surface with one leg extended out in front of you. Cross your other leg over the extended one so that the foot of your crossed leg is touching your extended leg's knee. Bring your opposite side elbow over to the crossed leg and make contact with your thigh. Using your elbow, twist your body and push away from your elbow/thigh. Move back until you feel resistance, then hold for 10-30 seconds. Switch to other side and repeat.

Knee to chest: Lie on your back with your legs fully extended out in front of you. Then, bend one knee and bring it towards your chest. Use both hands to grab the bent leg under the thigh just above the back of your knee and pull your thigh towards your chest. Hold for 10-30 seconds.

Butterfly: Sit on a flat surface with your knees bent. Place the bottoms of your feet together and hold them in place by grabbing onto your ankles. Hold for 10-30 seconds and repeat.

Hurdler's stretch: Sit on a flat surface with one leg extended and the other bent with your foot on the extended leg's knee. Similar to the toe touch, extend your arms out in front of you until you feel resistance, then stop and hold for 15-20 seconds. Repeat twice for each leg.

Calf stretch: While standing upright, place your hands up against a wall. Bend one knee forward while extending the other knee back. When you feel resistance, stop and hold for 15-20 seconds. Repeat twice for each leg.

Child's pose: Sit on your knees and place your forehead on the floor with your feet pointing out behind you. Extend your arms by your sides, palms facing up. Hold the position for 10-15 breaths. Repeat as desired.

Cat and camel: On all fours with your torso parallel to the floor, arch your back up and then slowly lower. Be sure to keep your arms straight.

Presidential Physical Fitness Award

To earn this award, students must score at or above the 85th percentile on all five activities.
One idea for an award is an odometer since the cost is only a dollar or less.

Presidential Physical Fitness Award Standards for Boys

Age	Sit-Ups (# one min)	Push-Ups (#)	Shuttle Run (seconds)	V-Sit Reach (inches)
6	22	7	13.3	+1.0
7	28	8	12.8	+1.0
8	31	9	12.2	+0.5
9	32	12	11.9	+1.0
10	35	14	11.5	+1.0
11	37	15	11.1	+1.0
12	40	18	10.6	+1.0

Presidential Physical Fitness Award Standards for Girls

Age	Sit-Ups (# one min)	Push-Ups (#)	Shuttle Run (seconds)	V-Sit Reach (inches)
6	23	6	13.8	+2.5
7	25	8	13.2	+2.0
8	29	9	12.9	+2.0
9	30	12	12.5	+2.0
10	30	13	12.1	+3.0
11	32	11	11.5	+3.0
12	35	10	11.3	+3.5

Shuttle Run

This activity measures speed and agility. Testing:

- Mark two parallel lines 30 feet apart and place two blocks of wood or similar objects behind one of the lines.
- Students start behind opposite line. On the signal "Ready? Go!" the student runs to the blocks, picks one up, runs back to the starting line, places the block behind the line, runs back and picks up the second block, and runs back across starting line.

Tips

Be sure the participants understand the importance of running through the finish line. Participants should perform this activity on a gym floor or other favorable surface.

Rules

Blocks should not be thrown across the lines. Scores are recorded to the nearest tenth of a second.

V-sit Reach (or Sit and Reach)

This activity measures flexibility of the lower back and hamstrings. Here's what you do:

- A straight line two feet long is marked on the floor as the baseline.
- A measuring line four feet long is drawn perpendicular to the midpoint of the baseline extending two feet on each side and marked off in half-inches. The point where the baseline and measuring line intersect is the "0" point.
- Student removes shoes and sits on the floor with measuring line between legs and soles of feet placed immediately behind baseline, heels 8-12 inches apart.
- With hands on top of each other, palms down, student places them on the measuring line.
- With legs held flat by a partner, the student slowly reaches forward as far as possible, keeping fingers on the measuring line and feet flexed.
- After three practice tries, the student holds the fourth reach for three seconds while that distance is recorded.

Tips

Participants are most flexible after a warm-up run. Best results may occur immediately after performing the endurance run.

Rules

Legs must remain straight with soles of feet held perpendicular to the floor (feet flexed). Students should be encouraged to reach slowly rather than bounce while stretching. Scores, recorded to the nearest half inch, are read as plus scores for reaches beyond baseline, minus scores for reaches behind baseline.

Sit and Reach Testing

Here's what you do:

- You'll need a specially constructed box with a measuring scale marked in centimeters, with 23 centimeters at the level of the feet.
- The student removes shoes and sits on floor with knees fully extended, feet shoulder-width apart and soles of the feet held flat against the end of the box.
- With hands on top of each other, palms down, and legs held flat, the student reaches along the measuring line as far as possible. After three practice reaches, the fourth reach is held while the distance is recorded.

Tips

Participants are most flexible after a warm-up run. Best results may occur immediately after performing the endurance run.

Rules

Legs must remain straight, soles of feet against box and fingertips of both hands should reach evenly along measuring line. Scores are recorded to the nearest centimeter.

Constructing a Sit and Reach Box

- Using any sturdy wood or comparable material (3/4" plywood is recommended), cut the following pieces: two pieces of 12" x 12", two pieces of 12" x 10", and one piece of 12" x 21".
- Assemble the pieces using nails or screws and wood glue.
- Inscribe the top panel with 1-centimeter gradations. It is crucial that the 23-centimeter line be exactly in line with the vertical plane against which the subject's feet will be placed.
- Cover the apparatus with two coats of polyurethane sealer or shellac.
- For convenience, you can make a handle by cutting a 1" x 3" hole in the top panel.

https://www.presidentschallenge.org/tools-resources/docs/getfit.pdf (2015, pages 9-20)

Appendix 3
Jeopardy Questions and Answers

1. Identify laminated fruits and vegetables.

2. What is real food?
   - Real food is picked from the ground.

3. Name 5 real foods?
   - Celery, spinach, cauliflower, cabbage, beets

4. What is the definition of processed food?
   - Processed food is machine-made using non-picked foods.

5. Name 5 processed foods
   - Burgers, hotdogs, chips, cookies, candies

6. What is a healthy snack?
   - Nuts, fruits, smoothie, banana chips, trail mix

7. What does obesity mean?
   - Obesity is when you have too much body fat

8. How can obesity be prevented?
   - By eating healthy real food, exercising, and sleeping well

9. What are the food fundamentals?
   - Water, fiber, protein, carbohydrates, fats, and vitamins

10. When you are thirsty, what is the best thing to drink?
    - Water

11. How much water should you drink a day?
    - Half your body weight in ounces. (If you weigh 80 pounds, drink 40 ounces/ 5 glasses of water)

12. How much of your body is made up of water?
    - 70%

13. What are foods that grow during the fall?
    - Squash, pumpkin, apple

14. Name a red fruit or vegetable.
    - Cherries, cranberries, strawberries, tomatoes, red pepper

15. What is the benefit of red fruits and vegetables?
    - Healthy heart

16. Name a yellow fruit.
    - Pineapple, banana

17. What are the benefits of orange and yellow vegetables and fruits?
    - Protection from some types of cancer; improve night sight vision; keep skin/teeth/bones healthy.

18. Name a green vegetable.
    - Spinach, cabbage, peas, broccoli, green beans

71

19.   What are the benefits of green vegetables?
- Good for bones, teeth, eyes, and preventing diseases such as heart diseases and diabetes

20.   Name a blue or purple fruit or vegetable.
- Plums, eggplant, raisins, prunes, blueberries, blackberries

21.   What are the benefits of blue and purple fruits and vegetables?
- Improve memory; reduce diseases such as cancer, heart diseases and Alzheimer's

22.   What does organic mean?
- Organic means food from the ground without chemicals.

23.   How much sugar should someone your age eat a day to be healthy?
- 3 teaspoons

24.   How much sugar does the average American child your age eat a day?
- 21 teaspoons or a half cup

25.   What happens when you eat and drink too much sugar?
- Hyper and diabetes

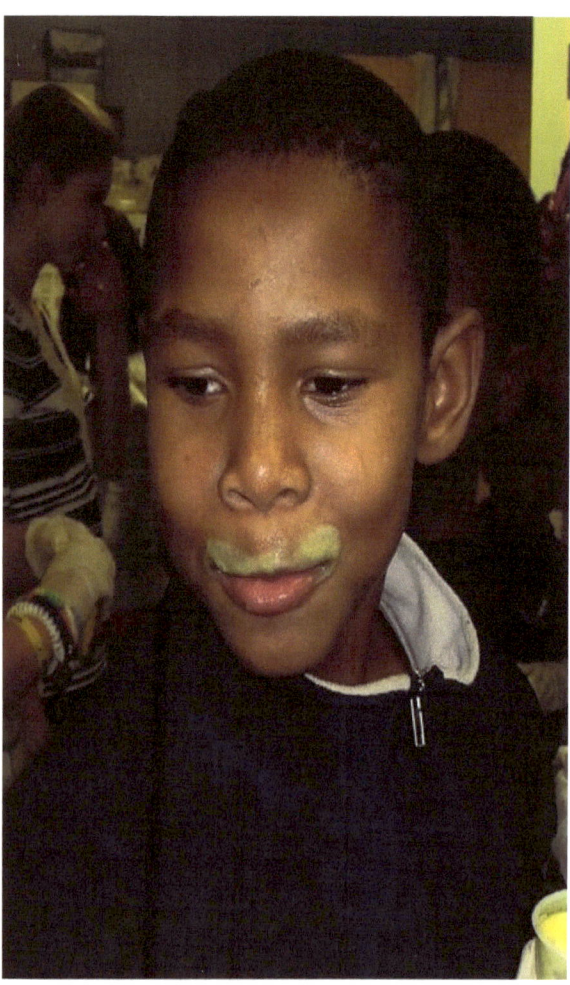

Appendix 4
Real Kids Real Food Curriculum
Ten Week Sessions - Introducing New Children Each Session

A. Introduction
1. What is Real Food? – Ninja Smoothies
2. Eating A Rainbow – Guacamole and Veggies
3. Eat Local and Seasonal – Apple Sauce
4. Field Trip to Farm
5. History and Benefits of Bananas – Banana Almond Butter Ice Cream

B. What's on Your Plate?
1. Fabulous Fiber – Cheezy Kale Chips
2. Good, Bad, and Ugly Fat – Real Trail Mix
3. An Awesome Fruit: Avocado – Kale Avocado Salad
4. Sugar Shock – Apple Crisp
5. Artificial vs. Natural Sweeteners – Carob Fruit Smoothie
6. Labeling and Nutrition – Sweet Potato Corn Chowder Soup
7. Art Changing Back to Earth – Fruit Art

C. Under the Hood: The Human Machine
1. Immune System – Sweet Orange Salad
2. The Digestive System – Eggless "Egg" Salad Sandwiches
3. Stress Free Kids – Sweet Potato Chips

D. Growing
1. The Life Cycle of a Plant (Photosynthesis) – Cinnamon Apple Chips
2. When Do Seeds Grow? (Seasons) – Ants on a Log
3. Soil Comparison (sandy, clay, composted) – Spinach, Banana, Strawberry Smoothie
4. Indoor Sprouting – Sprouted Hummus with Dehydrated Crackers
5. April Showers (Water) – Create Your Own Juices
6. Transplanting to the Outside Garden – Veggie Burgers
7. Caring for our Garden: Scavenger Hunt – Lemon Italian Ice

E. Holidays
1. Healthy Halloween – Witches Fingers
2. Thanksgiving – Pumpkin Pie
3. Festive Preparation and Gift Box – Truffles and Stuffed Dates
4. Holiday Party for Parents – Avocado Carob Mousse, Linguine Zucchini with Marinara Sauce and Apple Crisp
5. New Year, New You: Natural vs. Processed Foods - Eggless "Egg" Salad
6. Valentine's Day – Chocolate Macaroons
7. St. Patrick's Day – Green Smoothie